THE NEW
HOSPITAL
SUPERVISOR

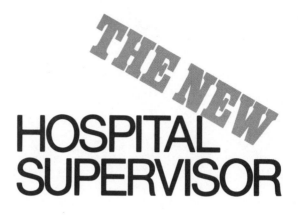

THE NEW
HOSPITAL SUPERVISOR

Nancy L. Diekelmann, R.N., M.S.
Assistant Professor
University of Wisconsin
School of Nursing

Martin M. Broadwell
Resources for Education and Management, Inc.

Cartoons by Johnny Sajem

ADDISON-WESLEY PUBLISHING COMPANY, INC.

Reading, Massachusetts • Menlo Park, California
Don Mills, Ontario • Wokingham, England • Amsterdam
Sydney • Singapore • Tokyo • Mexico City • Bogotá
Santiago • San Juan

Dedicated to A.S.H.E.T.

The American Society of Health Manpower, Education and Training

Foreword

The new supervisor has one of the most difficult jobs in the entire spectrum of hospital management. The first time he, or she, assumes responsibility not only for the people doing the job, but—directly or indirectly—for patient care, it can be an awesome feeling. Moreover, the new supervisor must start right in performing tasks that may be unfamiliar and may take years to learn to do well. The problems are complex, many-faceted, and sometimes indefinable—but the new supervisor is expected to deal with them all and handle them well.

No book will prepare someone adequately for that first day, but this book should offer some basic help. It will not solve all of the problems that come up during the first few days, or weeks, but our intention is to offer a place to start looking for answers. That is not to say that this will be a collection of theories. It won't be. There is very little theory here, though there is a practical application of many theories. People do not act theoretically; neither can they be supervised theoretically. The new supervisor has gone too far to be satisfied with just theories, no matter how good they are or how practical they have proven to be. What he or she wants to know is, "What do I do right now, with this problem?" Our purpose has been to help the new supervisor avoid making the same mistakes that have been made many times before by others. We won't guarantee no mistakes, but at least we want to offer the opportunity to make new ones.

Unit I deals with the reactions, feelings, and attitudes people usually experience in their new role as a supervisor; the loneliness involved in moving from one circle of coworkers to another; the frustrations that accompany setting old skills aside and learning new ones; and the worry, doubt, and just plain difficulty involved in having to see oneself and others in a different perspective. These are all basic problems that happen to most people and are hard to talk about, but they have to be dealt with before someone can feel comfortable with the new job.

Unit II focuses on the new skills the new supervisor will need. Since for the most part he or she is *unskilled* in the new job, the new supervisor tends to do whatever seems to be *natural*. Unfortunately, most of the needed skills do not come to us as natural gifts—we have to learn them.

Unit III, the last unit, deals with the new activities that go with being a supervisor, things like interviewing, writing reports, and running a meeting. This final section will attempt to suggest ways that the new supervisor can prepare for this part of the job.

With the economic pressures now being brought to bear on health-care institutions, and the rising costs of in-service education or hospital-wide training programs, it is imperative for new supervisors to assume some of the responsibility for seeking out information that will help them in a new role. If this book is used as a guide rather than as a handbook of rules, it should help the new supervisor to cope better and feel better in the new position. Hopefully, he or she will learn that what seems strange or perplexing or disillusioning at first is primarily a matter of learning some additional skills.

Decatur, Georgia   M.M.B.
Madison, Wisconsin   N.D.
November 1976

Acknowl

edgments

I would like to express my gratitude to all who helped me with this book. For their time given in assisting in the adaptation of this book, I wish to thank: Despina G. Demetriades, Director of Learning Resources Center, Gaston Memorial Hospital, Gastonia, North Carolina; Henry LaParo, Director, Training and Personnel Development, New York University Medical Center, New York; and Angela Milligan, R.N., B.A., Director, Health Education Consortium, Sardis, Mississippi. For their time given to reviewing the original manuscript, I wish to thank Martin J. Cregg, Director of Training and Employee Development, Western Health Management Services, Inc., Los Angeles, California; and Joyce Godwin, Personnel Director, Presbyterian Hospital Center, Albuquerque, New Mexico.

A special thanks to Raymond T. Bedwell, Jr., Director, Human Resources Development, St. Joseph's Hospital, Milwaukee, Wisconsin for his contributions to this book. And to Rose Lee Kennedy, Society Director, the American Society of Health Manpower, Education and Training, American Hospital Association, my sincere thanks and appreciation. Rose Kennedy breathed life into this project and was responsible for guiding me and supporting me in this sometimes seemingly impossible task.

To Alan Filley, Professor, Graduate School of Business, University of Wisconsin, my sincere thanks for his support and help provided in preparing this manuscript.

To my father, Lyle R. Poole, Jr., for his help and insightful examples while I was preparing this manuscript, my love and appreciation. To Robert Schuster for his patience and expertise in editing the manuscript, my sincere thanks. And to my husband, John, most thanks for his encouragement and unconditional love.

N.D.

Many have helped in my writing efforts, but few have offered more encouragement than Cathy Horat and Janice "Hamburger" McDonald. Both also exhibit those qualities we're suggesting for good health-care supervision. A special vote of thanks, too, for Dave Crissman and Bob McClure who allowed me to gain valuable experience and insight through training many supervisors with the Center for Disease Control.

M.M.B.

Contents

Unit I

ATTITUDES AND FEELINGS

Chapter 1

You

It's hard to explain what it's like being a supervisor to someone who has never had the experience. The first day on the job brings with it a lot of emotions that nonsupervisors probably never imagine—feelings like frustration, anxiety, regret, and loneliness. And these feelings don't just go away. A lot of new supervisors tell themselves that they were better off before being promoted, because at least they knew where they stood with the old job. Nevertheless, the job can be rewarding—ask any supervisor who's been around for a few years.

The question is, why is it sometimes so tough? And how do you know whether or not you're going to be happy with it? You have to understand that becoming a supervisor creates some major changes for you. Not only does the title change, but so too do one's loyalties, one's responsibilities, and even one's co-workers. With all of these changes, it's not unusual to feel disillusioned. In fact, it's normal.

A few years ago, one individual was promoted and became a supervisor in the engineering department of a large hospital. He'd been there fifteen years, and he was a fast, skilled, reliable worker—just the sort of employee you'd like to have working as a supervisor. Two weeks after beginning his new job, he found himself riding the members of his old crew, even though

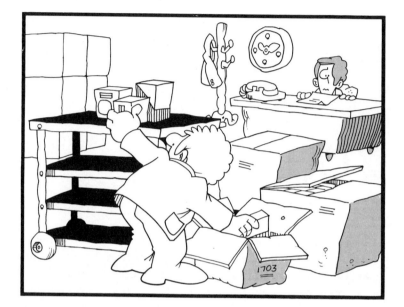

they were getting the work done. He wasn't happy with himself, and neither was the crew, obviously. The problem was, he was thoroughly frustrated. After all those years spent developing special skills and feeling responsible for certain jobs, suddenly it was *his* job to see that someone *else* did the work.

This happens all the time. The change from being one of several staff members to being the supervisor requires some important adjustments. Accepting the fact that someone else is going to be doing your old job while you watch is by no means the only or even the easiest adjustment a new supervisor has to make.

Let's look at another example. Ruth had always taken a lot of pride in working as a medical technologist. It was satisfying, rewarding work for her. Suddenly, after being promoted to supervisor in her own department, she found herself feeling that maybe it wasn't such terrific work after all—that maybe she'd made a mistake. The problem was that for the first time Ruth was being called on to do a job she had never been trained to do. How many lab techs, nurses, housekeepers, radiologists, or secretaries have ever had any training in supervising others? She was frustrated, because she knew she had the qualifications for the job—she just hadn't been trained for it.

Being a supervisor can be satisfying, but supervisors are not born—they have to learn the management skills necessary for being good supervisors. The difference between the person who is unhappy as a supervisor and the person who finds it rewarding is that the man or woman who is happy with it has worked hard at developing the skills he or she needs to use every day. The odds are that you, like almost everyone else, will start out feeling a little anxious in your new position. You'll probably remember the sessions you and the rest of the staff used to have around the coffee pot, when you really used to let the old supervisor have it behind his or her back. Those sessions have a way of catching up with you. You're the supervisor now, but the sessions haven't stopped—you're just on the other end of the conversation. Your anxiety is real, just as Ruth's frustration was. It gets in the way of your performance and satisfaction, but those kinds of feelings tend to go away as you gain the skills needed to deal with your new position.

You have to begin by preparing yourself to have an open mind. Becoming a supervisor changes things, including the way you have to look at things. It changes your perspective; you have to look at a bigger picture. For instance, although it doesn't take the human element out of your work, it does put other elements in—so you have more factors to consider when you make decisions. Let's say that Jill, a nurse on one of your units, comes in red-eyed and obviously has a problem. As the story unfolds, it looks something like this. She and her husband haven't been married very long, and this morning they had an argument. Her husband lost his temper and said some pretty terrible things. Jill has asked for time off to go home and pack before her husband gets there. The truth is, you can't afford to let her go—even without pay—because of the heavy patient load. As distraught as she is, there's no telling how she will react when you tell her she can't go. She's waiting now for an answer and needs it immediately so she can call her mother. What are you going to do?

The problem is real and important. As a supervisor, you are expected to make the right decisions. Suppose you let Jill go. Where will you draw the line the next time someone wants a few hours off? More importantly, how will her absence affect the patient care your unit provides? But, on the other hand, suppose you don't let her go. How well will she function the rest of the day, and what will your decision do to the morale of the unit?

Obviously, there aren't any clear-cut rules. Each situation has to be handled individually. A basic principle is to treat your staff as you would want to be treated, remembering that they are human beings with real problems and feelings. But there are problems even with a rule as general as that. You may not really be sure how you would like to be treated in a similar situation. And knowing what you do about work scheduling and a balanced budget means that you might want to be treated differently from those who don't know about these things. And suppose you do decide that Jill is a human being—so what? It's a nice thought, but what do you do with her problems now that she's become a human being? What do you do about fulfilling your direct or indirect responsibility for patient care in the hospital?

This may sound like a heartless question, but it really isn't. It just means that being a supervisor changes things for you. As it gives you more factors to consider, it also gives you the right and the opportunity to make decisions that were not yours before. Service and, ultimately, patient care become important now; and all these other things are part of providing that very important service. This doesn't make you any less interested in people. In fact, it makes you more interested in them, but in a different way. Patients have been entrusted to you—in a sense—and you have an obligation to see that they receive proper care.

Another feeling common to new supervisors is loneliness. The supervisor's position didn't seem too bad when *you* were part of the staff and *someone else* was the supervisor. You may remember yourself saying, "Supervisors have it made. We do all the work, and they get all the credit, the money, and the office!" The job looked easy then, but somehow it doesn't look that way now. Jill or Donna, Emory or Clinton even look different now. You know that they haven't changed, and you haven't changed, so what has changed? The JOB, your responsibility, your viewpoint—and let's face it—your loyalties have all changed. Whether you like it or not, the people working for you don't see you the same way now. And you can't afford to see them the same way either.

A few supervisors maintain their old relationships by telling the old gang that nothing has changed. They continue to go on break with them, eat lunch with them, gripe with them, criticize the hospital and knock the administrator with them, and still get the work done and handle disciplinary problems. But few successful supervisors have done this: there are plenty of failures to show that this is a dangerous route to take. Being "one of the gang" is nice, and it's all right too—but you can't give up being the supervisor just to remain a pal. Some of the people you work with may not be able to accept you as both a friend and a supervisor, so you may have to forego lunch with your old crew. You may find that some people, hoping to gain an advantage over someone else, try to use a coffee break to get the "lowdown" on what's happening in your department. You may choose to avoid that type of conversation, or you may have to announce that in your new role you would prefer that this type of topic not be discussed. You may feel that some people who were warm and friendly to you before seem quiet and withdrawn now and are uncomfortable around you. Any of these situations can lead to feelings of loneliness.

The important thing to realize is that now you are a member of a new gang. You have to give up some of the pleasures of being part of the old gang and accept your position as a supervisor. You now belong to a gang composed of other supervisors. You don't have to associate with them, but you do have to communicate with them on their level (which is your level, too). You may feel uncomfortable with this new gang for a while, but eventually you will feel a part of them.

What really has changed then? Your responsibility, your outlook, and, of course, your job! Will the feelings of frustration that you experience because you are not trained for the job of being supervisor, even though you are qualified, persist? The answer is that by reading this book you are already taking a step toward reducing that frustration. You are seeking out information about how to become a better supervisor that you can apply to your own situation. Your feelings of anxiety and nervousness will also begin to decrease as you handle more problems like Jill's and begin to develop confidence in yourself. And the loneliness? It can begin to go away if you think of the group that works for you as a team, and if you think that you must stick together and perform as a unit to meet the objectives of the hospital. But remember, even though you will work as one, *you* must be the leader. You must set the pattern of leadership by letting them be a part of the goal-setting. You must lead by giving them as much authority as possible, so they can do their job with a minimum of interference from you. And you must see that they develop their full potential and that their needs are met. But you must do these things as the *supervisor*, not as one of them.

THOUGHT QUESTIONS

1. As a new supervisor, how would you explain your new job to others in the department in which you work? How does the job differ from the position you held just before you were appointed supervisor?

2. Since it is so difficult to give up being a "doer" and assume the duties of a supervisor, what ways do you see to help a newly appointed supervisor stay out of this trap? What ways have worked best for you?

3. As a newly promoted supervisor, how do you explain your new job to others in the department with whom you've been working all these months?

4. What can you do or say that will help them to see that your role has changed from "worker" to supervisor?

Chapter 2

Your Staff

You may notice that the people working for you seem anxious to make a good impression during your first few days as a supervisor. You'll probably get the feeling that they're putting their best foot forward, trying to please you. And more than likely, you'll find yourself trying hard to be the perfect supervisor. This kind of special behavior is called the *honeymoon* period between a staff and its new supervisor; each party is worried about what the other is going to think and is trying to look as good as possible. It occurs because everyone is anxious and there isn't a great deal of *trust* built up as yet.

Because your staff wants to trust you, you'll find that this honeymoon period quickly gives way to a period of *testing* in which they'll be watching you carefully to see how you react in certain situations. Trust develops only after someone tests someone else, and the staff will be looking on to see what happens when someone does something wrong. Will you be tolerant and tell the person who made the error to forget it, or will you blow your stack and embarrass this person in front of everyone? What will it be like when there is a rush job to be done? Will you be the kind of supervisor who puts the screws on tight, or will you just relax and not worry about deadlines? What will happen when other departments interfere with your

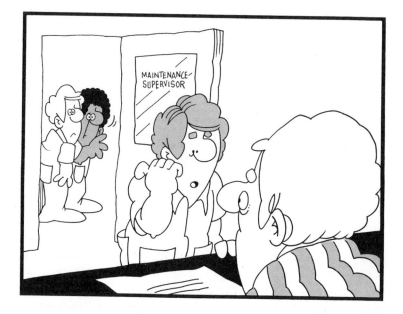

activities or don't do their part of the job? Will you stand up
for your rights, or will you let them run all over you? Your staff
needs to know these things about you before they can really
trust you, and they will be anxious about you until their questions are answered.

As a new supervisor, what does this mean for you? Let's
say that one of the housekeepers who works for you comes
to you early one morning and reports that yesterday two
workers who were supposed to help clean the linen rooms were
two hours late in getting back from lunch. You are expected to
"do something about it!" Let's say too that the two workers in
question have done outstanding work for you since you became supervisor. It is necessary for you to set limits on the behavior of your staff, but it is also important for you not to
respond on hearsay. Indeed, this informant may be testing you
to see how much a person can get away with.

As a new supervisor you should be prepared for this testing period. Frequently when a staff "tests" its supervisor, the supervisor feels as though he or she is doing a poor job. The temptation is to "act-out" how you feel. If you're angry at the staff for taking a long lunch hour, you may be tempted to assign them twice the usual amount of work instead of dealing with the problem. A supervisor may interpret the staff's long lunch hour as an indication of dislike or lack of respect, and may therefore try to prove by punishing them that he or she is *in charge* and should be respected.

It would be better for you to anticipate this testing period and be prepared for it, because testing is both normal and necessary. It is a means of developing trust. Your staff will know they can trust you when under difficult situations you show yourself to be consistent, honest, and concerned about them as people. The Housekeeping Supervisor, in our example, must be prepared for such testing situations and learn not to react with hostility and anger. The staff needs to see how the supervisor will react to this type of situation. Will he or she act on "second hand" information? Or ignore the situation? Are long lunch hours all right? Will he or she be punitive? Will he or she be fair and consistent with the staff?

When the staff is allowed to test you, your staff members will quickly develop a working relationship with you that is marked by trust. When this happens, their testing will stop. Absenteeism, being late, failing to follow directions, challenging orders, and abusing privileges are all testing behaviors that will go away once trust is established. A good supervisor encourages the trust of the staff by being consistent, fair, and concerned. Even someone who is known to the staff is going to be tested when he or she becomes a supervisor, and should know that there will be days when he or she will be tested by everyone. That kind of day can make even the best of supervisors question his or her ability to handle the job, and it may be helpful for you to spend some time with someone in the hospital training program or perhaps an older supervisor who can help you see that what you are experiencing is normal.

You will learn that one of the strange things about being a supervisor is that it is possible for the people working under you to love and hate you at the same time. Perhaps these terms are too strong, but they identify the problems brought about by the phenomenon of "ambivalence." This simply means that because you represent two different things to the staff person, it is possible for him or her to feel two different ways about you. As the supervisor, you represent authority—you tell people what to do and what not to do and hence pose a threat to their satisfaction. But as supervisor you also represent your subordinates' means of getting ahead, getting a raise, solving problems, being recognized, or being told how to do things more easily; thus, you offer real security. You are at once a comfort and a threat, and subordinates can both like and dislike you. This is reflected in their reactions to the way in which you give them assignments. If you just give them assignments without any directions, they complain because you haven't explained how you want the job done. If you give them instructions, they are apt to complain that you're looking over their shoulders all the time and won't let them do anything on their own. Again, your job as a supervisor is to recognize that this phenomenon of ambivalence exists, and to look for ways of using it to your advantage.

Often you may find yourself in the peculiar situation of apparently having to defend the authority that goes with your position. Very early in the game, you have to realize that there is nothing wrong with being a supervisor. Because new supervisors usually feel pretty insecure, they may feel a need to apologize for it or defend it, but every organization and every institution at almost any level needs someone in charge. For whatever reason, you, the new supervisor, are the person in that situation, and it's up to you to act the part. As a matter of fact, if you find yourself trying to defend your job, it is probably a good indication that you are still insecure in it.

Interestingly enough, while you may try to hide the fact or avoid it, the staff never really forgets that you are the supervisor. Whether or not you act as though it is your choice, they still know it no matter what you do. All that this means is that you should get the work done by being the supervisor, not by trying to be a friend or a buddy, or by trying to *bribe* the staff into doing what they are being *paid* to do. The problems of supervision arise *not* because you are the supervisor, but either because you don't act like one or because you exploit the job. While you do have the right to be a supervisor, you have no right to use that fact as the only means of getting the work done. You can't demand that the staff respect you, and even though you can get the work done for a while by demanding it, sooner or later that kind of action breeds disrespect and will return to haunt you. The staff will wait until they find you in a vulnerable position, and then, when the chips are down, they won't support you. So, during the beginning of your new experience as a supervisor, it is wise to act somewhere between the two extremes of trying to hide the fact of being a supervisor and exploiting it.

Whether you like it or not, you still have to depend on the staff to accomplish the long-range goals of the hospital. You can only do a limited amount yourself (and the more work you do, the poorer job of supervision you're doing). Sooner or later, you must get the work done through the people the hospital has given you to do it with, which is why your attitude toward these people is so important. You may think you don't have enough people or the right people or enough time for training, but it's still up to you as a supervisor to get the work done with the people you have at this time and under these conditions.

This brings up another thought. These are the people who—to a large degree—can make you or break you as supervisor. Your ability to use their skills, to motivate them to perform, and to get them to think and do the way the hospital wants are the things you will be rated on when appraisal time rolls around. So their performance will have a direct and important bearing on your rating as a supervisor.

Finally, you have an obligation to develop your staff because it is from their ranks that your job, like others, must be filled. The way you train, use, and treat your staff will determine whether or not the hospital has enough properly trained people to replace you and others like you when you move on to better things. While it may be difficult for new supervisors to think of developing skills in their staffs so that they may some day take their places, it is an indictment of a supervisor if he or she fails to develop anyone who is capable of handling much, if not all, of the work when he or she is out of the office or moved to another assignment.

THOUGHT QUESTIONS

1. You have just been promoted to supervisor. How would you treat one of your staff who has been your close friend during your years at the hospital?

2. As the new supervisor, you feel the need to "size up" your employees to help you know them better. What approach would you use to do this? What would you look for, and what do you want to know about them? What do you want them to know about you?

3. How do you learn to trust someone? What kinds of things do you do to get someone to trust you?

4. If you were the close friend mentioned in Question 1, how would you want your new boss to treat you?

Chapter 3

Your Department Head

As a new supervisor, you will have to develop a working relationship with your department head just as your staff must with you. More than likely, you will find yourself experiencing the same behaviors and feelings that you see in your staff. You may experience a brief honeymoon period, but it will quickly be followed by concerns that most new supervisors have in common, such as: What kind of boss will your department head be? How will he or she react when you make a mistake? How much can you trust this individual? How concerned is he or she about you as an individual? It is perfectly normal for you to ask yourself these questions, because you need answers to them before you can feel that you can trust and have a comfortable working relationship with this person. As a result, you may find yourself "testing" the department head, just as your staff may test you. The answers to your questions will come out of the interactions you have with this individual, and as your concerns begin to be answered, a feeling of trust will develop.

It might be helpful for you, as you begin to settle into your relationship with your department head and go through this process, to realize that he or she has a perspective of the hos-

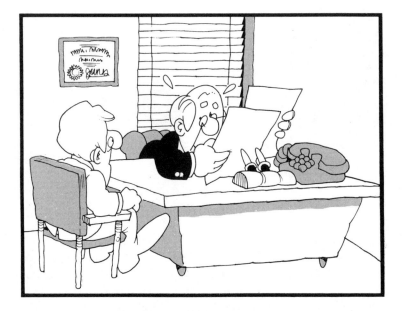

pital and its administration that is inherently different from
yours as a supervisor. Having responsibilities different from
yours, he or she sees less of the day-to-day activity of the hospital than you do. It is your position, not the department
head's, to deal with the daily problems and demands of your
staff and their duties. Therefore, he or she is less currently informed about those types of issues than you are. At the same
time, you see less of the total hospital picture than he or she
does, since issues of policy, major departmental budgetary
problems, and long-range goals are all his or her immediate
responsibilities. The point is that you will see things
differently from the way the department head does, not just
now as you are taking up your new responsibilities, but day in
and day out for as long as you have supervisory responsibilities. You will have to learn to live with the problems and
frustrations that can create.

Remember that your department head is human and is prone to the same types of feelings, pressures, and needs as you are. He or she experiences insecurity, anxiety, anger, and defensiveness just as you do. He or she too has worries about home, family, money, chances for promotion, relationship with the boss, and whether or not he or she is doing a good job. Your relationship may be more rewarding if you can maintain this perspective of your department head as a fellow human being.

As a new supervisor you are likely to experience several common feelings with regard to your department head that seem to reflect on your personality. One of these is that it may sometimes appear as though he or she is not really interested in you or that he or she is not concerned with your problems. Imagine, however, that one of your staff members comes to you with a problem just after you have been asked to produce a major report within a short period of time. Very likely you would have very little interest in your staff member's problems just at that moment, and more than likely he or she would feel personally neglected, being in no position to appreciate the pressures you felt. We said earlier that as a new supervisor you would have to broaden your horizon, but broad as yours must be, your department head has to consider areas that you do not have to consider. It is likely that his or her apparent lack of interest in your concerns will be related to problems that you may not be aware of, rather than to any particular attitude toward you.

Another feeling you may experience is a hesitancy to do a good job, because you may feel that good work will only make your department head look good. Of course this is true. When you as a supervisor do well, it does make the department head look good, since he or she works through you just as you work through your staff. But your good work also makes you look good. If he or she occasionally takes credit for what you have done, remember that you may inadvertently take credit for your staff's work at some time. The department head makes mistakes just as you do. The important thing is that it is to everyone's advantage for you to function as well as possible in your new role.

Finally, you ought to recognize that you as a supervisor have some responsibilities toward your department head. You need to keep this individual informed about what is going on in your department; he or she is responsible for making decisions which should be based on data provided by you. It is particularly important for you to represent your staff accurately to the department head. Supervisors occasionally forget to mention the positive things their staffs are doing and tend to focus on the problems which need the most attention. You must keep the department head informed about all aspects of your staff, both positive and negative, so that he or she has an accurate picture of your division. He or she may not necessarily agree with or support your desires for your staff, but remember that he or she has broader concerns than you do and that it may be impossible to reward your staff as you would like.

Remember too that your boss is one step removed from your staff and that if you do not provide complete and accurate information he or she will have to make decisions based on inadequate information. Consider the case of the new Blood Bank Supervisor, who was concerned about the performance of her new technician for over three weeks. She shared this concern with her department head, who suggested that if the technician was not able to function at a higher level, he should not be kept beyond the probationary period. The supervisor was glad she had informed her department head of the problem and felt more secure about it, since she was in agreement with the decision. A month later, however, when the probationary period was over, the department head asked the supervisor if she was prepared to discharge the technician. At this point, the supervisor realized that she had neglected to inform him that the technician had been showing steady improvement and that she was now reluctant about letting him go. As the discussion continued, the supervisor learned that one position in the lab had to be eliminated, and since the department head had anticipated the technician's release, he had told the administrative staff that it would be all right to eliminate that position. This is a perfect example of why your department head needs to be kept informed of what is happening with your staff. You need to develop enough confidence in your department head to trust him or her with complete, accurate information about your decision.

THOUGHT QUESTIONS

1. Can you think of an example where a problem was seen one way by your department head or his or her boss and a totally different way by you or some other member of the department? Can you explain the reason for these different interpretations?

2. Knowing what you do about your department head's job, how can you (as a supervisor and as a subordinate) help him or her to do a better job?

3. Even though you and your boss are both supervisory people, how do *your* supervisory responsibilities differ from his or her supervisory responsibilities?

4. As a supervisor you must sometimes explain and promote policies and procedures which you personally do not endorse. How do you handle such a situation with the department head? How do you handle these situations with your staff?

5. How do you find out what your department head wants to know about the work and people you supervise? What kinds of things does he or she want to know?

Chapter 4

Your Fellow Supervisors

Having accepted the new responsibilities and rewards that go with being a supervisor, you must exchange membership in your old work group for membership in a new group made up of your fellow supervisors. You may find yourself experiencing a variety of feelings ranging from jealousy and competitiveness to anger and insecurity as a consequence of this change. These are all normal feelings for the new member of any group to experience. Nevertheless, it is particularly important that you learn to understand and control them.

Characteristic of hospitals is the dependence one department has on another; that is, the dependence each supervisor has on all other supervisors. The life-and-death matters treated by the hospital require that you be able to work with your fellow supervisors; and while it may at first be difficult to adjust to your new group and to work comfortably with other supervisors, remember that you were promoted in part because of your department head's confidence in your ability to cooperate.

Perhaps the first if not the greatest stumbling block in your relationship with other supervisors will be jealousy concerning the relationships they have with the department head.

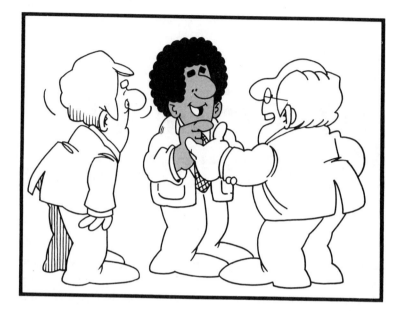

Most new supervisors experience this feeling. You may find
yourself being overly sensitive to the amount of time your boss
spends with another supervisor in your department. You may
overreact to any signs that indicate he or she may like another
supervisor better than you. You may even be tempted to tell
the department head something that will make you look good
at another supervisor's expense.

Obviously, this is unacceptable, immature adult behavior;
but it occurs frequently when people feel insecure. Initially,
new supervisors are insecure because they do not know the
head of the department or their fellow supervisors well enough.
As they work with them and get to know them personally and
professionally, these feelings generally go away. As you begin
to feel more relaxed and comfortable in your relationships with
your new group, your initial jealousy should give way to more
productive and rewarding feelings.

Still, there may always be differences between you and other supervisors. Certainly there will always be things they can do that you cannot do as well. The opposite is also true; you have special skills that other supervisors do not have. While such differences are inevitable, they do occasionally lead to feelings of jealousy that can be longer lasting and more harmful than those mentioned earlier. Clearly, it is essential that you not let these feelings interfere with the services offered by the hospital. It may help if you focus on skills you have which others do not have. By being aware of your feelings and their causes, you may be able to control them.

It should go without saying that you should never allow your jealousy to lead you to take advantage of an opportunity to "show up" another supervisor. You might someday need his or her support, or you might even be in the same position, so it is as important for your own sake as it is for that of the hospital that you control your emotions and avoid "one-upping" another supervisor.

A greater stumbling block to harmony between supervisors may be loyalty. New supervisors usually try to instill a sense of loyalty in their staffs, and obviously loyalty can be a good thing. It makes your staff feel as though they have a common goal, and it encourages them to work together as a group. It may sometimes spur them to greater effort than they might otherwise have given.

On the other hand, loyalty can be counterproductive. While loyalty can encourage a staff to improve the patient care it is providing, it may also mean that one nursing unit might refuse to send staff nurses as relief when another unit is short-staffed. People often find it easier to be loyal to a small group than to a large, less homogeneous group, and consequently they develop stronger feelings for the immediate work group than for the hospital. At times these feelings of loyalty are so strong that individuals may even refuse a promotion to another group. Such loyalty, when it interferes with the overall patient-care goals of the hospital, is undesirable.

The answer to learning to work with other supervisors is free, open, and honest communication devoid of jealousy and exaggerated competition. The interdependence of departments in the hospital means that you need to know what is going on in other departments with other staffs and their supervisors. If you want to be able to rely on their communicativeness and cooperation, you must also be willing to share with them what is happening in your department with your staff.

As a supervisor, you need to work together with the other supervisors to *anticipate* conflicts and problems before they have developed too far to be stopped or corrected. To this end, you need to get into the habit of providing as much information as possible to those who work with you. Do not rely solely on verbal communication. Write memos and notes when appropriate to tell other supervisors what you might be doing that could affect their operations. When you do so, they and their staffs will be better prepared to contribute to solutions of your problems or completion of your projects.

Finally, staff members occasionally come into conflict with members of other departments. When this happens, you as a supervisor must proceed calmly by gathering facts and encouraging communication. You are not obliged to start an interdepartmental fight whenever one of your people has a problem with someone outside your staff. That implies building the wrong kind of loyalty. You must not even pretend that you are going to get this "straightened out once and for all," since that implies hostilities between you and another supervisor. In the long run, your staff will respect you more if you provide a smooth working environment for them. Your ability to get along with other departments and other supervisors is important if you are to be able to offer a constructive atmosphere to them; and consequently your ability to work with others is a sign of your skill as a supervisor.

THOUGHT QUESTIONS

1. As the new Admitting Supervisor, you have an idea for solving a hospital-wide problem—the availability of wheelchairs. But to implement it requires help and cooperation from the other supervisors. How would you approach one of them for help? What would you say?

2. How would you tell another supervisor about a project you have in mind, to be sure he or she doesn't feel you are trying to criticize or make him or her look bad to the department head?

3. What kind of an approach would you take to solving a problem which appears to be largely the fault of another department?

4. What kinds of activities would you use to *maintain* and reinforce good relations with the other supervisors in the hospital?

Unit II

SUPERVISORY SKILLS

Chapter 5

Communi-
cating

We have been talking about your reactions and the reactions of others to your new role as supervisor. This chapter will look at your communication problems and the process of communication.

Every one of us functions both verbally and nonverbally in a very complex society. In order to survive, we have had to become skillful in the way we communicate with others, so communication skills are something we all possess to some degree. Nevertheless, every new situation brings with it the opportunity and the need to reexamine the forces affecting the communication process. As a new supervisor, you will have to rely heavily on your ability to communicate effectively and efficiently with your staff. As a hospital supervisor, you may encounter special communication problems.

An understanding of what makes communication difficult in the hospital, the principles of communication, the factors affecting communication, and common communication problems will be helpful to you in your new role. This chapter will look at this process of communication in a way that will allow you to apply the information to your own staff and your particular situation, rather than dealing in general terms with communication skills themselves.

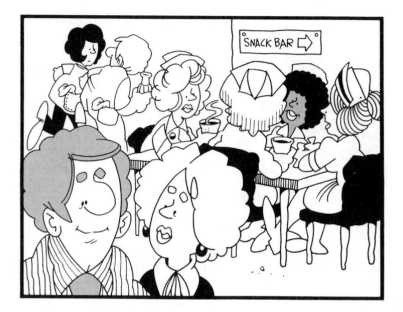

WHAT MAKES COMMUNICATION
IN A HOSPITAL DIFFICULT?

All of us are familiar with the common lunchtime routine in which the people who spend their day working together tend to eat together. The same principle applies to hospital-wide meetings, breaks, and even fire drills. Nurses tend to sit with other nurses, particularly those from the same ward. Housekeepers tend to talk with other housekeepers. Lab techs tend to socialize with other lab techs. All of these examples illustrate a basic rule: people communicate most freely and most often with people they know.

This presents a particular problem in the hospital. Hospitals are divided into numerous, specialized units of employees, all of them separated by geographic distance. Many times it is impossible to know everyone, simply because you are so rarely in close contact with each other.

Secondly, each group has its own rules, values, and special meanings. Normally, members of one group are to some degree unaware of the rules and values of other groups. This not only creates a sense of psychological distance between departments, it also presents some very practical barriers to good communication.

Finally, when something occurs that requires communication, it is usually important to notify certain people first and others later. The problem is knowing with whom to communicate, at what time, and with what priority. Because of the complexity of activity that goes on in the hospital, the answers may change from one situation to the next.

PRINCIPLES OF COMMUNICATION

While the hospital is inherently a complex situation in which to communicate, there are several fundamental principles underlying communication that can be helpful to you in maximizing your ability to communicate both with your staff and with other departments. The following principles have been supported through communications research.[1]

1. *Within a hospital, as in any other organization, people have certain forces acting upon them to communicate with those who help them achieve their aims and other forces acting to discourage communication with those who will not assist or may retard their accomplishments.* An example of this can be seen by observing who it is that people turn to when they have questions, or when they have a "minute" to talk. Usually it is someone who is identified as being supportive and in a position to help rather than someone who is hostile, unhelpful, or unknowledgeable.

[1]Jay M. Jackson, Ph.D.: "Lines of Communication," in *Management for Nurses—A Multidisciplinary Approach*, ed. Sandra Stone, et. al. (St. Louis: The C.V. Mosby Company, 1976), pp. 49–57.

Supervisors who have not been visibly supportive of their staffs may find that staff members who are particularly anxious to be promoted go directly to the head of the department instead of to them with their comments and suggestions. This leads not only to embarrassment, but also to a very real breakdown in intradepartmental communications.

2. *People direct their communication to those who make them feel more secure and gratify their needs and away from those who threaten them, make them feel anxious, and in general provide an unrewarding experience.* Research has shown that staff members respond positively to supervisors whom they trust and believe are genuinely interested in them. Every supervisor should behave in such a way that the staff feels that he or she is considerate and accessible.

When a supervisor opens the mail during a supervisory meeting or during the hour that has been set aside for meeting with the staff, he or she is destroying the opportunity for effective communication. Fellow supervisors, or staff, may justifiably interpret this behavior as an indication that they are less important than the mail is; and this may make them anxious and perhaps angry.

3. *Persons in an organization are always communicating as if they were trying to improve their position.* This may not be a conscious behavior. Sometimes staff members are reluctant to ask their supervisor for help when they need it for fear that it might look as though they were admitting some inadequacy. Supervisors often delete from their conversations with their staff any references to their own mistakes. Some employees, especially those with extensive skills or experience, resent close supervision, since it implies that their power and prestige are less than they want them to be. Therefore, these individuals tend not to communicate fully and openly. Finally, individuals tend to

communicate with people who may be in a position to increase their status, power, or authority. If by using open communication individuals decrease their status, then genuine problems or constructive suggestions will go without acknowledgement and the department will be run less efficiently than it could be.

FACTORS AFFECTING COMMUNICATION

From these basic principles, it is possible to summarize some of the underlying factors in your relationships with your staff and with other departments that may contribute to the success of your communication efforts.

The effect of any particular communication in the hospital will depend largely upon the prior feelings and attitudes that the people who are involved have toward one another. It is important to encourage communication so that people understand your actions and expectations. Research has shown that when people like each other increased communication makes their observations and perceptions of each other more accurate. On the other hand, when they dislike each other increased communication does not result in increased positive feelings. When you do not like someone, you are reluctant to reveal yourself, and no amount of communication will reduce your feeling of dislike.

A second factor that affects communication is the relationship between the supervisor and his or her staff and how adequately this relationship satisfies the staff's needs. We have already talked about the importance of trust and how trust is developed, and *now* we need to look at trust from the perspective of its effect on communication. When there is a trust relationship between the staff and the supervisor, staff members are not afraid to reveal and share their true feelings, but it is difficult for a staff to trust a supervisor who is *unclear* and *inconsistent* in his or her dealings with them.

A final factor affecting communication is the amount of support that staff members feel they get from their peer group. When staff people feel that they are part of a group, they are more likely to disagree with the supervisor and to make counterproposals, but they will be less defensive and more problem-oriented. The peer group is important because it helps staff people validate their ideas or opinions. When communication is directed to a group as a whole rather than to isolated individuals, it is more likely that an accurate transfer of information will be achieved.

COMMUNICATION PROBLEMS

Let us summarize, then, how these principles and your information about the factors affecting communication can play a part in some of the common communication problems you may experience. When communication problems do occur, they are usually symptomatic of something else. The following are four of the common reasons for communication problems.

1. Lack of Trust

When trust exists between a supervisor and the staff, fellow supervisors, or the department head, content is more freely communicated and recipients more accurately perceive the sender's message. When trust does not exist, people are relectant to express themselves and are more likely to misinterpret information that is given to them.

2. Lack of Common Goals and Agreement

When people have different goals and value systems, it is especially important to create mutual understanding about needs and motives. People initiate and spread rumors—which create confusion, anxiety, and distrust—when they are unclear about what is happening or when they are powerless to affect their own destinies. Passing on a rumor is a means of expressing and alleviating anxiety about the subject of the rumor.

3. Lack of Understanding about the Social Structure of the Organization

It is important to understand the issues of work, authority, prestige, and status relationships in the hospital. Not knowing whom to notify first when a problem arises and not understanding the ground rules of communication—such as whether it is best to notify all individuals of changes at the same time or if for some reason the supervisors must be notified first—can lead to a breakdown in communication due to resentment and hostility.

4. Unfair Distribution of Rewards

It is important to distribute rewards fairly, so that people's needs are met and so that they are motivated to contribute to the overall objectives of the hospital. Communication can be severely restricted if staff members feel that they will not receive credit for their contributions.

THOUGHT QUESTIONS

1. You arrive one morning to find that your staff has heard a rumor that you are being transferred to another department and that they will have their second new supervisor in six weeks. Based on information presented in this chapter, what factors can you suggest that might account for this type of gossip? What could you do to prevent it from spreading or occurring again?

2. The new bookkeeper consistently goes to the supervisor with questions, even though they can be answered more easily and quickly by other members of the staff. Using information offered in this chapter, what explanation for this behavior can you suggest? As the supervisor, what would you do to help the bookkeeper begin communicating with the other workers?

3. As a new supervisor, you begin noticing that no one on your staff ever consults Nurse Smith for information, even though she has been working for the hospital for 16 years. In attempting to get to know her better, you find that she tries to avoid contact with you. Drawing from the information in this chapter, what reasons can you offer explaining why your staff may not be communicating with her? What reasons can you suggest to explain why she avoids communicating with you, the new supervisor?

Chapter 6

Motivating

Why do people work? Studies answering this question have found that people work for a vast variety of reasons, but that almost invariably satisfaction is a reason for staying on a job. People want to find satisfaction in their work. Jobs offering appreciable salary increases along with poorer working conditions are very often passed over for jobs that offer greater non-monetary benefits. Satisfaction, and thus motivation, is affected by a variety of factors, such as the link between performance and rewards and knowing what a good job is.

It is important, then, for you as a supervisor to understand what it is that provides people with satisfaction if you want to motivate your staff to continue or improve their level of work. It is very clear that satisfied employees have less absenteeism and turnover than do dissatisfied workers.

SATISFACTION AND MOTIVATION

Individuals find different things satisfying. Some people describe jobs as satisfying if they offer fairness, peace of mind, stimulation, pleasant sensations, and absence of guilt or anger. Others find satisfaction when there is a sense of achievement, responsibility, and advancement. The variety is endless.

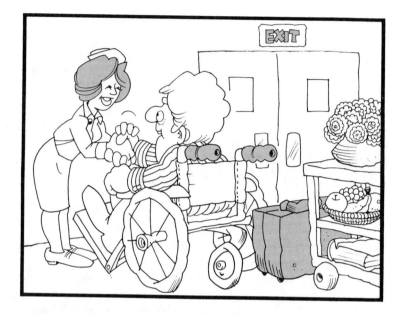

People do those things which they *think* lead to satisfaction and avoid those things which they *think* lead to dissatisfaction. The emphasis here on "think" is deliberate. Something thought to be desirable may not in fact lead to satisfaction, but an individual is motivated by what he or she thinks will lead to satisfaction whether or not it indeed does. On the other hand, something one person desires you as a supervisor may not desire. A lab supervisor may not find it particularly gratifying to be mentioned in the hospital paper, but the new lab technician might find it very exciting if he or she were trained in the hospital and still had a number of friends there.

The lesson is that if you want to motivate people to increase their performance, it is important for you to find out what appears to lead to satisfaction for them, since they will do those things which seem to offer satisfaction. How people define satisfaction is an individual matter. What is important is that you as supervisor understand something about how to provide it for your staff.

FACTORS THAT AFFECT MOTIVATION

Now let us look at the specific factors that affect motivation as people seek satisfaction in their work.

The first factor is the answer to the question: *What is the likelihood that if I try to do this type of work I will be able to succeed?* We all have seen excellent employees who, when promoted to jobs in which they say they lack skills, soon find themselves unable to perform well and becoming frustrated, angry, and finally apathetic. One of the things that motivates people is the estimation that if they try to do something they will be able to do it.

If as a new supervisor you want to increase motivation in your staff, you might consider demonstrating to them that they can do their jobs at a high level of performance. Try to increase their self-esteem at every opportunity. It is not only important that you show them they can do the job, it is also important for you to provide them with the praise and other rewards necessary to raise their self-esteem.

Occasionally, it may be impossible for you to demonstrate to an employee that he or she can do the job well. It may be that the individual simply doesn't have the needed skills and is unable to learn them. In cases like this, it is important that you suggest a change in job so that the employee can find a position in which he or she can succeed. This may sound harsh, but it is to the employee's benefit as well as yours to make it possible for him or her to perform at the highest level possible. It is much better to change the job than to try changing the employee.

Do I know what a good job is? The employee cannot be motivated to perform well without knowing what constitutes good work. As a supervisor, you must ask yourself whether or not the job you expect someone to do is clearly defined. Does the employee know exactly what you expect? Have you taken the time to go over the details together to be sure he or she

understands? Does the employee know where his or her job
starts and someone else's ends? Are there gaps or overlaps in
assignments? These concerns do not just call for a job description, they require taking a comprehensive look at the work
responsibilities.

We have all heard the argument, "It's impossible to
describe the job exactly, hospitals are complicated places, and
there is no way to predict exactly what is going to happen." In
a sense, this is true. Emergencies do arise. But in another
sense, this is a "cop-out." To the best of your ability, you need
to look carefully at what your expectations of your staff are,
and you need to check them out with your employees to see if
they perceive their jobs in the same way you do.

Not only should staff members understand what their jobs
consist of, they also need to know what level of performance
you expect. If you demand a certain level of performance, it is
important that you discuss it with your employees and come to
an agreement about it. People tend to perform on a level that
they have agreed to.

**How clear is the connection between performance and out-
come?** In other words, is there a clear and visible link between good performance and rewards? Your staff will
quickly form an opinion as to whether or not good work pays
off. For example, if doing a good job means that they will be
promoted, they will be motivated to perform well. If, on the
other hand, they feel that no matter how hard they work only
your "friends" will get the promotions, then the odds are that
they will not be highly motivated.

As a new supervisor, you must be very careful about when
you give rewards, to whom you give them, and what they will
be. Rewards for good work are best given immediately, but be
very careful to reward only desired behavior. If you reward all
behavior ranging from average to excellent, you will encourage
average work. Be careful not to reward unacceptable behavior.
Routine or automatic rewards do not motivate people to per-

form at a high level. You must also try to discover what a reward would be for a particular employee. For some people, a reward means being praised in front of their peers. For others it may mean a written memo to the department head or an offer to pay for morning sweet rolls. It is important that you know your staff members well enough to be able to individualize the rewards you give, since if the outcome of good work is not something the individual values, he or she will not be motivated to perform at a higher level.

Finally, it is important to establish an open system of giving rewards. If promotions or salary increases are offered in an unpublished, closed system in which the employees are not aware of the criteria being used to evaluate them, you will not be encouraging motivation. The more that you are able to show and publicize for your staff the exact system you use to give rewards, the higher the motivation in your department is likely to be.

HOW TO INCREASE MOTIVATION

Considering these factors, then, what specifically can you do to increase the overall performance of your staff?

You might begin by employing the kind of person who values the rewards you can provide in your department. If you are unable to reward good work with money, you should avoid hiring people who are highly motivated by salary increases. If you can offer an attractive benefit system, or if you can acknowledge job performance through promotions, then the type of person you will want to hire is the one who is motivated by these rewards.

In terms of your current staff, you should begin by trying to determine what your employees regard as rewarding and make every effort to provide those types of rewards. You should be very careful to avoid generalizing. One staff person may perceive more responsibility as a reward, while another may regard it as simply "more work."

Occasionally, an individual's title is changed without a corresponding change in his or her job. This is not a reward, and as a supervisor you must be very sensitive to this type of problem. Giving a person *more* of the *same* type of work only enlarges the job, it does not enrich it.

Lastly, since it is impossible to satiate an individual's need for personal growth, you must provide your staff with continuing opportunities for growth. As long as people continue to learn and feel as though they personally are benefiting from their work, they will remain involved, satisfied, and motivated.

THOUGHT QUESTIONS

1. On the basis of information presented in this chapter, how would you answer a new supervisor who comes to you and asks, "How can I get my new aides to want to do a good job?"

2. Assume that you have met with several members of your staff to ask them to review your new procedures manual. Since the staff has a heavy work schedule, you have to ask them to do this on their own time. They respond by asking for a Saturday afternoon off for a picnic in return for their extra time. You are very short-staffed on weekends and cannot easily afford to give them the time they request. What would you do to assure their cooperation and maintain their motivation?

Chapter 7

Planning

As we have already seen, it is the job of supervisors to get work done through other people. They are doing their best work when they deal with the problems of getting the job accomplished, rather than doing the work themselves. While new supervisors are directly responsible for the workers and their performance, they are still not supposed to do the work themselves. (Of course, emergencies arise, but we're talking about the normal supervisory activities).

THE SUPERVISOR AS A MANAGER

Some people make a distinction between "supervisor" and "manager." For our purposes in this and the following chapters we will talk about the supervisor's job of managing. Since the usual definition of a manager is "one who gets the job done through people," we won't do any harm if we use the terms interchangeably. The supervisor has certain managing responsibilities. We will want to see what that means to the new supervisor.

Everyone above the worker or specialist level has some managing to do. The only difference between the first-line supervisor and the head of the hospital is the scope and responsibility of the managing assignments. Basically, every manager, whether he or she is the hospital administrator, department manager, head nurse, or unit supervisor, has four managing functions to perform:

- planning,
- organizing,
- directing, and
- controlling.

While all supervisors are involved in all of these functions, the extent to which they perform each of them usually depends on their level in the hospital. For instance, the administrator would probably spend most of his or her time planning and organizing, while the first-line supervisor or head nurse should devote most of his or her time to directing and controlling the activities of the staff. Since all supervisors participate in all of these functions, let's see what they really mean to the new supervisor.

PLANNING

First, let's be sure we understand something about all of these functions. Each is something that is done along with, and as a part of, the job. While we should learn each as a skill and be aware of the fact that we are doing it, we shouldn't be scared off because it has a fancy name. The chances are pretty good we'll do some of each one, whether on purpose or by accident. So when we talk about planning, we're talking about the everyday job—how it's done, what will be done tomorrow, where we hope to go from there.

Planning is by far the most important of all the activities we've listed because everything else results from it. It is, simply, the means by which supervisors decide in what direction they want the group to go. The process can be done carefully or it can be haphazard. The interesting thing is that even doing nothing will still produce a result! The hospital will still exist, tomorrow will still come, and the employees will do something, right or wrong. Most experts agree that planning is the most important of all the functions.

It is much harder to correct the results of poor planning than to do it correctly in the first place. The results of poor planning can be pretty disastrous, and, unfortunately for new supervisors, they usually show up more quickly for them than for the higher administration. When top administration makes a mistake in planning, it sometimes takes many months or even years for it to come to light. When the first-line supervisor makes poor plans, it sometimes is only a matter of hours before the results are known. For instance, if the administrator decides to put more time and effort into a campaign to increase contributions to the hospital building fund or needed capital equipment purchases, it could take a year to see whether the campaign was a success. If a team leader plans staffing needs incorrectly and has too many people off during a peak time of admissions, the resulting ineffective or inefficient patient service will be evident before the day is over.

HOW AND WHAT TO PLAN

How do we as supervisors plan our work? Obviously we want to consider whatever alternatives are available to us and select the best one, all things considered. Too often, supervisors think of planning as deciding to do—or not to do—one certain thing. Good planning always takes into consideration all of the possible alternatives, weighs them carefully, then selects the one with the most merit. There is a caution here, though: Don't try to find the perfect solution, or the one that has no draw-

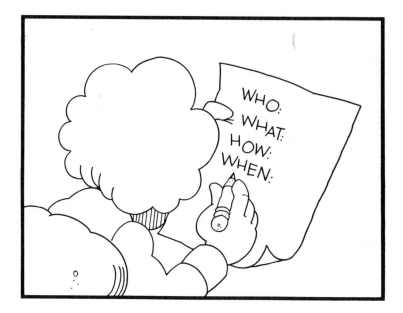

backs. There seldom is such a plan. In fact, we may have to settle for the plan with the fewest drawbacks, because none of the plans is completely satisfactory. Because we are in the people business, and our daily work deals unpredictably with patients' lives and health, you may think we cannot apply these planning ideas to health care. Not true! Because we know crises will occur, we can and should plan for them by planning work to include both the routine jobs and some quantity of the unexpected events.

We form our plans by making four basic decisions:

1. What is to be done?
2. Who is to do it?
3. How is it to be done?
4. When is it to be done?

Now let's take these one at a time and see how they fit into the day-to-day job.

1. What Is to Be Done?

We should have this definitely in mind before we go on to any of the other questions. For example, it isn't enough to decide that we are going to give our staff more training, then go out and find someone to do the training. We must first decide exactly what training is needed, how much we can do ourselves, how much can be done by somebody else, and how much can just be left undone. If we aren't careful, we'll find ourselves trying to carry out plans that weren't very definite to start with, the results being a lot of muddling around trying to make something work that didn't have a very good start. So the rule here is to be sure that we know exactly where it is we're going before we start to go there. It isn't necessary to write all our plans down, but it sometimes helps us understand what we are going to do if we make a positive statement on a note pad of just exactly what we plan. Of course, the plan may change as we go along, but at least we have something to change. Otherwise we'll end up making our plans as we go, changing those, repeating our errors, and in general botching it all up.

2. Who Is to Do It?

Part of planning is to determine whether this is a project for the whole staff on each shift, for just a few of them, or for one individual. If it is a one-time job, there is a great advantage in having only one or a few people work on the project. It's easier to keep up with a special project if only a few people are involved and less training time will be required. On the other hand, if the work is the kind that will continue to be a part of the responsibility of our work group, then our planning should include deciding how soon we want everyone to learn the new work.

There is an important training note here: if we aren't careful, we may let a job just gradually slip into being. No one is ever really trained for it, but finally everyone is doing it—and probably not very well. We may have it in mind that one of these days we'll do the training, but we keep putting it off until a more convenient time—which never comes. A basic fact to remember about training is that like everything else on the job it must be planned for. Left alone, it will not happen. The good supervisor plans for it to happen!

3. How Is It to Be Done?

Once a goal or objective has been decided (and agreed) on, we still have to decide how it's going to be met. This decision has to be considered at every level, but especially at the first level. Policies about the work will be set at higher level. The decisions about the actual work are usually made at that point in the hospital where the work is to be carried on, hence the first-level supervision. (The decision may not always be made here because the supervisor gives up some authority to the boss. The head nurse then complains about lack of authority to carry out the job, when in reality the authority wasn't used when he or she did have it.)

Policy setting is sometimes done unconsciously, because we can set policy by doing nothing. If we don't come up with firm policies on matters such as overtime, safety, time off, vacations, shift rotation, promotions, or appraisals, precedents will begin to set the policies for us. If we intend to do a job without adding staff, we may be setting a policy for more overtime toward the end of the job!

4. When Is It to Be Done?

The final question to be decided has to do with one of the most important ingredients in successful planning—time. While the obvious conclusion is that the completion date is the most important consideration in time, this is only part of the story. No deadline is missed all of a sudden. Long-range plans usually fall through because of poor short-range planning. As first-level supervisors, we are seldom directly involved in the long-range objectives of the hospital, but we are often very much involved in the short-range plans. So meeting these short-range objectives is the most important "time" aspect of our role in planning.

WHO'S WATCHING THE CLOCK?

Something that should concern us all as new supervisors is the fact that since the administration is interested in the "big picture" (i.e., the long-range objectives), they usually aren't watching the short-range objectives as closely. This means they may do no more than get an occasional progress report, always keeping an eye toward the final completion date. If we first-line supervisors aren't careful, we may be the only ones watching the short-range dates. We can be sure a lot of people will be looking, though, when it's too late to do anything about it.

Sometimes at first-level we may have the illusion that everybody is watching everything, and that we're just insignificant cogs in a giant wheel. But once we've been trapped by this thinking, we're heading for trouble, especially with short-range plans. Even though everyone seems to be watching over our shoulder, they still expect us to watch the day-by-day progress of the work. For example, if the long-range objective is to reduce absenteeism, the administration will be concerned with quarterly, or perhaps monthly, reports, but we—and the other first-line supervisors—must worry about who shows up and who doesn't every day.

OBJECTIVES AND POLICY

Planning, then, is a function of management in which we are concerned with the future of the hospital in those operations for which we are responsible. In the process of planning, we decide where we are going and how we intend to get there. Usually, we call "where we are going" the objective and "how to get there" the policy. Some have compared this to a ship taking a trip. The objective is the destination of the ship, while policy is the course the ship must take to get there. In a sense, planning is the rudder steering the ship. The supervisor doing the planning controls the ship, and without planning the ship has no rudder.

While it won't be dealt with in detail in this chapter, we should learn quickly that the more we take our people into the planning effort, the more likely we are to reach the objective. Since we are more likely to be involved in short-term planning, we are setting short-term objectives, often with short-term policies. These may well be day-to-day type things that our people know as much about as we do. Getting them to assist in setting deadlines is a good way to get commitment to these deadlines also. Getting them to participate in laying the ground rules is a good way to motivate them to work according to these ground rules.

CONTROLLING

In the next chapter we'll talk in detail about the function of controlling. We need to mention it here because planning and controlling are very closely associated with each other. The supervisor controls according to the planning that has been done. For example, budgeting is a type of planning, but the budget itself is a control. While it is being prepared, the budget is part of the planning function. Once the operation is begun, it becomes part of the controlling function.

Other examples might be quality control or service standards. Determining the hospital's policies on quality or service is a basic part of planning. When those policies go into operation, they are actually controls. The importance of all of this is that we should be glad that budgets, standards, and controls exist, because it is through them that the desired end result is reached. They not only direct the way and tell us when we've reached the objective, but they give us a standard to measure against all along the way.

UNDERSTANDING THE PLAN

It's almost too obvious to mention, but no plan is very good if it isn't understood by those affected by it. The reason for mentioning this is that we tend to blame someone else when a plan begins to go awry. The first thing we should investigate is whether or not the planning included safeguards against misunderstanding the plan. Were the employees informed? How were they informed? Were they just told or did they get an opportunity to ask questions, seek additional information, and generally become familiar with what was expected of them?

This sounds like something pretty big that would only be done when some major operation is undertaken. Not so. The employees need to know what's expected of them even in a small, one-hour assignment. Remember, our people are more interested in the day-to-day activity than in the long-range operations, so it's the smaller things that are important at this level.

ORGANIZING

So far we've talked about only a part of what is necessary to set up the work. There is another function called *organizing* that plays a big part in getting us to the final objective we have set. Organizing is a pretty broad term and generally includes two things: the *structure* of the hospital we have set up to do the job and the *people* in this hospital. Since the administration usually handles the structure of the hospital, we'll look mostly at that part of organizing concerned with people. First, though, let's note that we aren't talking about something big and complicated when we use the word "hospital." We're simply talking about any group of people who have joined together to get something done that they couldn't get done by themselves. This fits the small work group in one unit as well as both rural and urban hospitals. And the same principles apply.

In Chapter 10 we will talk in detail about interviewing prospective employees, so we won't go into that here. However, since part of organizing includes staffing our own hospital, we should realize that when it comes time to fill a vacancy in our group we will be expected to do an interview. Also, since the prospective employee will be working in our hospital, we should look forward to meeting and finding out as much as possible about him or her. Most new supervisors, however, dread this particular phase of the job. A little knowledge of how to conduct the interview—and a little experience—should cause these fears to diminish considerably.

RIGHT PERSON—RIGHT JOB

The whole object of the staffing phase of organizing is to try to match up the potential of the employee with the requirements of the job. Unfortunately, we often find that through poor staffing we end up making ourselves and our employees miserable. Often we do a poor job of matching a staff member's skills and interests with the job, then blame the employee for poor performance. We should really blame ourselves for poor judgment!

Getting the right people to do the right job makes a lot of sense from a lot of standpoints. Obviously the employees have fewer frustrations, see they are useful to the hospital, and feel they have a chance to be recognized. As a result, they are most likely to be motivated to do their best and will be reasonably satisfied. From our standpoint as the supervisor, a lot of our problems are solved, because their motivation should reduce absenteeism and turnover and increase productivity. We will then have more time to handle other phases of our job. From the hospital's standpoint, it is not only getting services for wages paid, but is also getting a good picture of us in the process. When our people perform well, it naturally reflects favorably on us. Note, too, that a mismatch between employee and job can make all of these things come out unfavorably.

There is another phase of organizing that we will deal with in detail in Chapter 11, which is *training*. It isn't enough to try to match the individual and the job as well as possible. We must still make up the difference between the employee's present skills and the job requirements. This can best be done by training. Given enough time and patience, of course, employees will learn on their own. In fact, many do. But this is rarely the most efficient way or the most practical approach from the hospital's point of view. Not only do we need to have the employees know their job, we need to know they know how to do their work. Training gives us this knowledge, because we see that they have had an opportunity to learn the skill. If it's good training, we will see them actually demonstrating their proficiency. Then if they do not do their job properly, we look for some cause other than lack of training.

THOUGHT QUESTIONS

1. What parts of the job on a patient-care unit can be planned using the four decisions (what? who? where? when?) mentioned here?

2. How far down into the health-care work force should planning take place?

3. Many first-line health-care supervisors admittedly don't plan. Why is this so?

4. What convincing examples from your hospital can you give in which more or better planning would help get the job done?

5. What approaches can a supervisor use to get subordinate supervisory people to do more planning? How can he or she know that it is, in fact, being done?

Chapter 8

Directing

Any supervisor can view his or her job as one of getting the work done through other people. No matter how many or how few people he or she supervises, that's the job. Planning and organizing—discussed in Chapter 7—set the stage for the next two functions, *directing* and *controlling*. The best of plans and the best organization won't do the work. Only those under us can do it, and we must direct them in doing it, and control the efforts they put forth while doing it. In most cases, planning and organizing are done at higher levels in the hospital, while directing and controlling are done at the lower levels—usually at first levels. So, as new supervisors we must be doubly conscious of the functions of directing and controlling.

Of all the functions supervisors perform, by far the hardest is directing. Directing involves people and people are complex, unique, and often different from one day to the next. People's needs vary as do their ambitions; and as these things change, so does the way they react in given situations. This means that just about the time we have figured out how a certain person will react to certain things, he or she changes on us because of something we may not even know about (at home, at church, at the little league field, etc.) and now he or she reacts completely differently the next time we say or do something.

But the situation isn't hopeless. There are some common grounds on which people react pretty much the same way all the time, and even different people react the same way to certain things. This means that there are some things we can do that will give us a predictable result, even though we do it to people who are otherwise quite different from each other. Once we have found out these things we can build our "management philosophy" around them. Let's look at some of these things and see if we can't find a basis on which to act and react with our people.

FACETS OF DIRECTING

There are three facets of directing: leading, communicating, and motivating. Each is a skill, but each is hard to learn and even harder to define.

Leading

Let's discuss leadership first. What is leadership? Ask a dozen people, and you'll probably get a dozen different answers. It is a vague quality, but one that is recognizable in the people who have it. (More accurately, we can recognize the results of its presence, if not the quality itself.) Perhaps the easiest way to define it is to say that it is "the ability of a supervisor to inspire his or her subordinates to work hard to achieve the goals of the hospital." As we see, this is easy to measure, but hard to recognize as a specific thing that a supervisor does to get results.

One thing we know: the idea that leaders are born, not made, is out of date. All of us can be better supervisors than we are. There are things we can learn that will produce better results. There are skills of leadership that can be practiced, learned, and measured. There are, in fact, some characteristics that are shared by people who have been rated as good leaders, and we can develop these as we get more experience and training.

For example, successful leaders are usually considerate and have the ability to see the other person's point of view. They don't necessarily agree with it, nor do they give in to it, but they at least have some empathy for it. They are sensitive to the other person's problems; they know why the person feels the way he or she does. They know how what they say will be taken—how it will affect the individual. They probably know how the individual will react to certain things that are done, and when the reaction is different from what they expect, they may even be able to analyze why it's different. Perhaps most important: successful leaders don't just attribute every undesirable behavior to "bad attitude."

Another characteristic good leaders have is the ability to see themselves as others see them. We generally speak of this as self-awareness. Here again is the ability to see how what we do will influence others. We should know how what we say will sound from the other person's point of view. Will the other resent it, miss the point altogether, or agree with it in principle? Good leaders can predict the answer pretty closely. Good leaders will even know their own weaknesses and faults and try to build around them so they won't interfere with their performance or that of others under them. The important thing about seeing ourselves as others see us is that we are more likely to treat others fairly if we know they are reacting to something we have done or said, and especially if we know why they are reacting that way.

A third characteristic of successful leaders is the ability to treat staff members as their equals, to be accessible to the staff, to explain actions taken, to be responsive to suggestions, and to represent the needs of the staff to others.

Finally, they have characteristics relating to the ability to initiate structure, such as scheduling work to be done and making job assignments, insisting upon work at full capacity and criticizing poor work.

Communicating

In an earlier chapter we discussed the subject of communication in great depth, so we suggest that the reader go back and read this again to get a refresher on the subject, this time keeping in mind that effective communication is an important characteristic of leadership. There are a few points that need to be mentioned here, though, that were not mentioned earlier.

When we can get a specific message across to another person or a group in just the way we want it to get across, that's good communicating. Whether we are writing letters, speaking to groups or individuals, giving orders, or passing on policies, we haven't ended our responsibilities until the message is received and understood. Whenever we hear ourselves saying, "Don't you remember, I told you . . ." we can be sure we have just indicted ourselves as poor communicators. We have said to the receiver, "It's your problem, not mine!"

The best single measure of our ability to communicate is to see if what we said produced the results we were trying to get. After all, that's the usual reason for communicating, anyway—to get some kind of action. The best sign that the message has been transmitted successfully, then, is to see if the policy is being carried out, or the people are coming in on time, or the person is responding in a way to indicate that he or she really understands what has been said.

One final word about good communicating: it isn't an asset, it's a requirement of the job. Supervisors must accept the responsibility for what they communicate. They cannot leave it up to those on the receiving end. They cannot blame the staff for not getting the message; they must see that they get it even if it means doing the communicating all over again.

Motivating

In order to motivate our staff, we have to understand why people work in the first place, and what it is that makes them work harder or keeps them from working as hard as they can. At one time people worked just to stay alive—they worried about food, clothing, and shelter, and the safety of their families. These things don't motivate today's average worker because the needs have long since been met. But we still have certain social needs that must be met, and we are motivated when we see a chance to meet these needs. Many people are motivated to receive satisfaction from such things as recognition for personal achievement and the opportunity for personal responsibilities. For others, interesting work and advancement in the hospital provide motivation to perform at a high level.

On the other hand, certain areas can provide the employee with dissatisfaction which discourages motivation. These areas include unfair hospital policies, poor relationships with a supervisor, and unfair pay. Unsatisfying working conditions and poor technical supervision are also frequently areas of dissatisfaction for many people. Obviously some of these areas can be dealt with directly by the supervisor, while others are handled by the hospital administration.

In encouraging motivation in your staff, you should always try to increase a person's self-esteem. This is related to what we just said, in that people like to think that what they are doing is important and that they are good at doing the work. It's hard for any of us to get motivated over a job that has been downgraded and specified as not really amounting to much as far as the hospital is concerned. That's why people worry about titles, having their name on the door, or being in the official directory. They want people to know that they are important enough to the organization to be recognized for it. Such little things as putting name plates on desks or titles on name badges often will go a long way toward meeting these needs. But employees also want to feel that the other workers respect them for their ability to do the job. They want them to think that what they do is important, and they like to think that they are looked up to for their ability. When reprimands occur in front of others, or we put someone in an embarrassing position, we are destroying the self-esteem that is so important to the worker. That's the main reason that we are always told to "correct in private" and "approve in public."

In discussing these three points—leading, communicating, and motivating—we haven't meant to imply that we should "baby" the employee. It is just common sense to recognize that certain things cause the worker to work better, and that we should take advantage of these things. This is simply a calculated effort to get best results from the individuals who work for us. In a way, it isn't really much different from treating a fine piece of machinery with proper care and maintenance. It is our way of getting employees to work because they want to, not because they must. In the end, the results are better for the hospital and its patients, for the supervisor, and certainly for the employees themselves.

CONTROLLING

While directing is the most difficult function, controlling is perhaps the most critical. When we plan, organize, and direct, there is still the problem of controlling all of what we have planned, organized, and are directing. Without the proper controls, all the effort may be wasted. Essentially, the supervisor is controlling three things or a combination of them; namely, money, material, and people. The problem is that each is handled differently; each takes a different skill. We find it easier to budget money and materials because they are usually quite constant. Money will buy just so much and we have just so much money, so the decision is what to do with what we

have. But people aren't that easy to budget; they aren't all
alike, and even a single individual may show different qualities
from one time to another. While a dollar is a dollar, a worker
isn't a worker. Replace one secretary with another and things
can be quite different from when we had the first one. When we
start to budget (control) people, we have to take into consideration that they work at a different speed in the morning than in
the afternoon, and their attitudes and behavior may be a lot
different on Monday than on Friday, or on PM's and nights.

Controlling is most closely related with planning, which
simply says that we must have something to control. Often-
times we may find ourselves trying to control when we
actually have no plan to follow. A plan serves as the standard
against which we control, so without a plan we are doing some
guesswork with our controlling. For example, when we decide
in the middle of a project that it's taking too many supplies
and hours of effort and start to "control," we really aren't
measuring this against a preset standard (or plan), so it isn't
completely correct to say we are practicing the function of control. If we had planned correctly and started our controlling as
soon as the plan went into effect, things wouldn't have gone
out of control in the first place. A rule of thumb (which is not
really a rule but a guide) says that when we find ourselves
needing to take drastic action with people, materials, or
money, either the planning or the controlling stage broke down
somewhere. We generally think of controlling as consisting of
three steps:

1. Determining standards.

2. Measuring results against standards.

3. Taking remedial action as necessary.

As we have said, the plan is the standard, but here we are talking about something more specific. We are looking for the
answer to certain basic questions. We need to know who sets
the standards and how we will know that they are the stan-

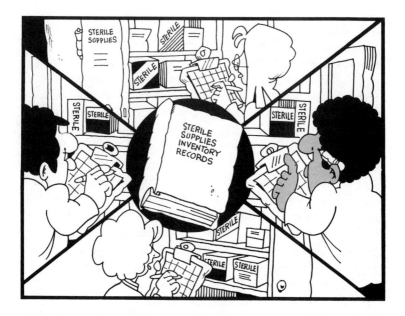

dards. The plan may or may not have specified how far off the standards we can get without being in trouble. That is information we must have; we cannot hope to control without it. Another thing we need to know about the standards is who will measure the results of our work and who will see the results of those measurements. Is there a quality-control person (like a system engineer or the infection-control officer) who reports to higher management, or do we have someone on our own staff who has been given partial responsibility for watching quality?

Of utmost importance is the question of what will be measured. Why is this particular thing being measured? Are we really getting valid information or are we just watching a meaningless figure? For example, do we fill out forms that tell how many bills are processed in the accounting office but fail to watch the cost of orienting the new employees or the amount spent in rearranging or redesigning offices? The point here is that we must be controlling the right things or the controlling effort will go for naught. Along the same line, we may find ourselves controlling something to death. If we have four people assigned to monitor the quantity of stock sterile supplies on the unit when our inventory records already show us this information, we are in fact "driving a tack with a sledge hammer." We sometimes discover ourselves overreacting to situations. The boss says to watch out for certain problems or expenditures, and we set up a control system much more complicated than is really needed. Long after the crisis is past, forms are still being filled out and reports being sent up the line. Once forms and reports come into being, it's very difficult to get rid of them. *Start them only under extreme need!*

What are some of the items which may be measured? Obviously we want to measure output of services. How long did it take to provide the X-ray service or to give a respiratory therapy treatment? How much did it cost? What was the final quality and how many treatments did we actually give? Then we need to look at expenses closely. When we measure expenses, we must measure all of them. Are we taking into account everything that is being charged to the particular job? Are we considering staff help, hidden costs, set up and cleanup time, and other costs that will eventually have to be included?

Another thing we must account for is the use of resources. Again we're talking about people, time, and money—but this time in a little different light. Here the question of measurement is one of efficient use. Are we doing a good job of matching people and jobs? Remember, it isn't necessarily proof of good supervision if the job gets done well. We must consider who's doing the job. If our people are capable of doing much more because of experience, education, training, or natural talent, we can't be too proud of the fact that the job is done well. The trick is to match ability and job requirements as closely as possible, then let the people grow out of their jobs as they develop. As supervisors we must constantly measure—at least in our minds—how well the employee is matched to the job, as well as whether he or she has outgrown it.

All of this is true for the other resources we have. Are we really getting the most out of our overtime? Are we doing some jobs that could be left undone or eliminated altogether, then using time and money on overtime to do essential things? We get trapped sometimes by saying that we have to go into overtime to do a very important job, failing to realize that we got into this situation simply because we failed to control our time properly. We spent valuable time at unimportant things, forcing ourselves into overtime. The same objection applies to using people on nonessential jobs or assignments when they could be doing things that must be done sooner or later. It's all right for everyone to pitch in and help when admissions are very heavy, but if this pitching in means that we must neglect other work that will get us behind schedule or cost us time and money later on, then we've made a bad decision.

USING THE BUDGET TO CONTROL

Perhaps the oldest and best control device we have is the budget. We complain about it and even wish we didn't have it, but we should be glad that there is something as rigid as the budget to guide us in our controlling. Very few hospitals could run very smoothly without a budget because it gives us one of the best standards we could have. It not only gives us something to measure our progress by, but also something at which to aim. As we constantly compare ourselves with the budget, we are also getting feedback on where we can expect to end up at the end of the budget period. Here is a means of measuring even the small parts of the job, because budgets are made up of parts. Good budgets are made up of accurate parts; bad budgets are made up of padded or "guesstimated" parts. This isn't the place to go into detail on the budget, but let's notice a thing or two about it. First of all, it is put together to let the administration know just how much money is needed and where the best places to spend it are. Good budget planning takes into account local needs, and those putting it together will solicit help from all levels in determining the best use of all the funds. The trouble comes when each level starts to be unrealistic about it's needs. When each unit, department, or service adds just a little, by the time the total budget is drawn up there is either too big a demand or the hospital finds itself looking for more money than it really needs. The fate of most budgets is that when this happens, someone at the top starts to whittle down the figure and everyone gets hurt. "But if I don't raise my figure, I'll get hurt, because they will probably make an across-the-board cut!" Even if this is so, that's a management decision and doesn't give us the right to pad our figures just because everyone else does. We shouldn't include anything we can't substantiate, because sooner or later we will have to account for what we have requested. If our figures won't stand the test, not only will the budget be cut, but our reputation as a supervisor will suffer. The wisest thing to do is to make a realistic budget, back it up with a good set of requirements, then let management wrestle with the problem of cutting it if they must. Later on, if the work isn't done because of budget problems (lack of money or people), we can show that we put in a legitimate request that got cut by someone else.

MEASURING RESULTS

Once we have determined the standards by which we are to control, we have to measure the results against these standards. Sometimes this measurement is routine—just a matter of seeing how many lab tests were run, how many pages were typed, how many patients were treated, and so forth, then reporting the obvious results in whatever manner is provided. But all of our evaluating isn't that obvious or that easy. Sometimes we find ourselves in situations in which there are so many contributing factors that we aren't quite sure just what the results mean. For instance, the operation may be too involved, as with complex team care on a rehabilitation floor, where many people and services are making different contributions to the end result. How can we measure in circumstances like this?

One of the best avenues open to us is the process known as sampling. There isn't anything complicated about it. It's just a means of looking at large or complicated services and getting reliable results without having to get a measurement on every detail and every person doing work in that effort. We simply look at a small, average sample and take the results to represent the entire operation. Another way to accomplish the same thing is to take one complete case or instance out of several, assuming that all the rest are like this one. Actually, with a little help, we can do a pretty good job of sampling and get very reliable results. Once we get in the habit of doing this, we are on the lookout for ways of getting true samples all of the time. We check the employee absentee list on random occasions and see if particular individuals or a particular number are absent. We spot-check three or four days in a row and see just how much time the employees are taking for break or when they are coming back from lunch or break. We look at patient complaints once a week for several weeks and see if anything is beginning to give trouble. These things are good indicators of just how well we are doing, and are good means of controlling.

When sampling doesn't seem to be a very good way of measuring the results, and the measuring seems to be too difficult to do on the whole operation, there is another way that may help. This is the simple matter of finding a substitute measurement. For example, we can look at such things as absenteeism or tardiness and get a good idea of what the morale is in the group. If turnover is high, this sometimes may be a good substitute measurement of the extent of job enrichment and training that are available. A look at previous records may be a good measure of motivation or employee morale in the work unit, providing other things are equal. The substitute may be a tangible means of measuring very intangible things, such as attitudes, job satisfaction, morale, etc.

Of course, when we are measuring one thing to look at something else, we'd better be sure the measure is accurate, which is true of any of our measurements. Even measuring such things as how well one clerk is doing compared to the other clerks in the office may not give meaningful results. If one person is typing simple records and the others are typing more complex material, such as complicated medical terms, a page count provides a poor indication of actual accomplishment. On the other hand, an individual doing the same simple job day-in and day-out may begin to show a high error rate because the job doesn't have sufficient variety in it. He or she may even come to envy those who have a more challenging job. If this clerk's accuracy was once high, the errors may indicate that he or she is getting less satisfaction than previously. It might be the same for an X-ray technician. We need to be careful in evaluating one technician against another because their patients may be entirely different. It's all right to measure efficiency by the number of radiographies a technician is taking, but only when we know how other technicians have done with like assignments. If one tech isn't doing well, have there been equipment breakdowns? Is he or she new and lacking experience? Does he or she really understand the new equipment? Has he or she been trained to use the new procedures and record forms? In other words, is our measurement really accurate in all respects? If so, then it becomes a good control device; if not, it becomes a dangerous tool to use in making decisions.

REMEDIAL ACTION

Controlling would be useless if it didn't include the final facet of control—taking remedial action when it is required. While controlling shouldn't be thought of in just these terms, it certainly includes this. When things are shown by our measuring processes to be running along smoothly, then we should be good enough supervisors to recognize this and leave things alone. But when the results show that the situation is getting out of hand or that we should really be doing better, then we need to know enough to step in and take some action. We may not be the ones to take the action, but we may be the ones to instigate it. As obvious as it seems, just knowing that something is wrong isn't enough; reporting it to the right people is important. If we have found that a problem exists somewhere on the unit, we should ask ourselves who really needs to know about it. The obvious answer should be someone who can do something about it. Whether it's an overtime problem, a union grievance, or what have you, telling the right person as soon as possible may head off a much more serious problem later on. When it comes to determining who the right person is, perhaps the worst thing we can do is to say, "It's not my problem." Remember, it's our problem as soon as we hear or know about it; and it's our problem until something is done about it, or someone else takes over the responsibility for it. When our department head says, "Okay, I'll take over now," then we have done all we can, even if we don't like what he or she is doing.

Another important part of notifying the right person at the right time is doing it in the right way. And that doesn't mean making a telephone call just at quitting time and giving only the bare details. If the person doesn't understand the importance of the problem, or misses some of the details, we've got to accept the responsibility for the poor results that come from improper control. The best approach is to put the problem in writing, which not only puts the information in permanent form but also provides a record that we spotted the weakness and made an effort to get it controlled. But this latter reason is secondary to the first one. It's no justification to report something just to protect ourselves. If this becomes our prime reason for acting, we aren't likely to do a very thorough job of reporting the facts; neither will we work at organizing our material, making sure what we say is clear, readable, etc.

Finally, let's repeat what was said earlier. It's a lot better to solve the problem ourselves than to pass it on to someone else. This means we must have the authority to take the necessary remedial action. It also means we may have to go through the entire planning, organizing, and directing functions all over again. If that's what the remedial action requires, being a good supervisor means doing it that way, rather than just closing our eyes to reality and going ahead toward eventual unsatisfactory results.

THOUGHT QUESTIONS

1. Some people say that today's "new worker" is different from the way we were when we started working in health care. Does your experience support that idea? Have attitudes toward working changed?

2. What are some good ways to control the work to be certain your coworkers continue to perform up to standard?

3. A good worker suddenly goes "sour." What reasons could there be for this sudden drop in output? How would you go about finding the causes in the work unit you supervise?

4. How much should you involve your workers in the efforts to control budget, materials, and manpower?

Chapter 9

Problem Solving

Problem solving, like most of the other things discussed thus far, is a skill. There are specific steps in the process which, when properly followed, pretty well guarantee success. The difficulty often comes when we start to look at the process, because the steps *sound* complicated. Actually, the process is simple and is the one we use most of the time in our personal decisions. When we consider buying a car, a house, or a boat, we go through these steps. We don't necessarily go through them *consciously*, but we deal with each of them nevertheless. As we discuss the steps, then, it's a good idea to think about how we use them in solving our everyday problems. If we already use the process, one might ask, why talk about it here? The reason is that we use the process or its steps on *big* problems, but not on the small problems that often can grow into big ones if they aren't handled correctly. Also, there seems to be some reason why we don't always make the application to the job, even though we use the ideas in our own affairs. (For example, while we realize that we quite often have to resort to buying things on credit—and in the process end up paying more money for them—we fail to see that the hospital we work for runs into the same problem; i.e., insufficient cash to buy now and save money later.)

We suggest you develop the habit of using the specific steps on small items until you automatically go through the steps in any problem situation. We will look at the steps, see how they work, give some examples, and leave it up to you to make the application on your own. Again, let's emphasize: the steps just sound complicated, they aren't really all that hard to understand and apply!

DEFINING THE PROBLEM

The first step in problem solving is to be sure we are attacking the *right problem*. Say an employee comes to us complaining of being tired of working on a certain job. If we take that at face value and start to solve that problem, we may find that we are working on the wrong problem, and maybe creating another. In reality, this employee may be fed up with us as a supervisor, or may have had about all he or she can take from an employee who works the same floor, or may be making more mistakes than he or she would like to because of insufficient training.

How do we know whether we are trying to solve the right problem? The best way is to do what the physician does when he or she looks at a patient—get all the symptoms together and see what kind of picture develops. This way we won't be treating just a symptom, but the real problem. Once we get the symptoms in we start to ask "What are the things that could produce these symptoms?" If employees are performing poorly, that may be a symptom of poor attitude, which may be a symptom of poor supervision or poor working conditions. Are there other signs, such as high turnover rates, absenteeism, tardiness, etc.? Are some of the employees performing all right while others aren't? Have these same employees performed better in times past? Only after we have satisfied ourselves with the answers to these questions can we be sure that we are dealing with the correct problem and not just a symptom. Once we are sure that we know what the problem is, it's a good idea to state it for our own clarification. "Reduce loss of start-up or processing time. Reduce the error rate. Increase the total overtime hours for the unit." Note that it's not the time to say, "Reduce the total overtime hours caused by poor work scheduling." This assumes that we already know the cause of the problem, which may be the case, but it's a good idea to get a few more facts before stating this. This brings us to the next step in the problem-solving process.

GATHERING INFORMATION

The information stage is an important one, but one that's often taken too lightly. After having spent so much time defining the problem, haven't we got enough information? No, not at this stage. We aren't ready to solve the problem yet. We must get as much information as we can, first to help us be sure we really are concerned with the right problem, then to help us pick up some ideas on how to solve the problem. Once we've gathered whatever facts seem to be available *in the time allowed us to look*, we take one last look and see if we really are on the right track. Have we discovered that every supervisor before us has had the same problem with the same employees on the same job? This doesn't make the problem go away, but it does change the complexion of the problem.

Notice that we said that we gather as many facts as time allows. One of the important decisions that the supervisor has to be able to make is when to stop looking and start solving. In other words, he or she must be able to recognize when further investigation would take more time and effort than the problem deserves. We might like to have attendance records going back for ten years, but if such information would take weeks of digging by a number of employees, we need to be able to measure its value against the cost of obtaining it. On the other hand, if the information is available right in the payroll files, we can't use the excuse, "It'll take too long to get the information." Note, again, we aren't looking for a solution yet, so the information we get should be gathered with an open mind. It would be wrong to obtain only that information that will help us prove a point, rather than solve the real problem. If we go into the problem-solving process with preconceived notions of what we are going to do anyway, then following specific procedures is just a useless exercise.

It is essential, during this information-gathering stage, that we get specific information, rather than generalities. We need to find out things like who or what, how many, how much, where, when, how long, etc. We will find that this kind of information is harder to get than general comments, but much more reliable in the long run. For example, it's not enough to have statements like "She's late all the time." We need to ask, "How many times in the last month?" We shouldn't accept information like "This floor-sweeping machine is costing us a fortune in repair bills." Such information will sink our argument one of these days. If we don't ask it, our boss might: "How much is a fortune?" Admittedly, generalities and opinions are much easier to get, and we probably make more friends when we ask their opinions instead of making them dig up *specific* information. But we are trying to solve a *specific* problem; hopefully, we are going to recommend that *specific* *actions* be taken. If all of this is based on just opinions, then we aren't likely to have the best solution available. By the way, when we're getting this information, we should make some kind of mental or written note on just how reliable the information really is. If some information is questionable, we should so note it, because later on we may find ourselves making decisions based on that information just as if it were completely reliable. If we know that there is some doubt as to the validity of the information, we'll treat it with caution later on. If not, we may forget and create a little grief for ourselves that could easily have been avoided.

FINDING THE CAUSE

The reason we have stressed so hard the fact that we aren't yet ready for the solution is that at this point we are ready to identify the *cause*. Only when we have found the cause can we select an appropriate solution. Using the information we have gathered, we look at all the possible causes. If we decide that the cause of the poor work output is the result of inadequate training, not poor materials, then we have some valuable data to use toward applying the proper solution. However, we may find that we will need more information or a different kind of information to get rid of the cause.

The difficult thing to remember is that causes aren't always easy to find. Rather than say that the cause isn't obvious, we should say that the cause that is obvious may not be the real problem. If we have a problem because one of the clerks in the admitting office is being too snippy with nurses on the units, the cause may not be a bad attitude; it may be that we haven't made the assignment completely clear and the clerk is protecting the job in the only way known—by keeping others away from it. Employees who are afraid that their jobs aren't as important as others will do their best to make it seem that way, even if it comes out as trying to make life miserable for other people: "I'm sorry, but I'm too busy to help right now," or "Did the supervisor tell you to handle that? That's my job and I don't want you messing it up." The cause may be poor supervision, poor definition of work responsibility, inadequate work, or several other things. But if we've gathered enough information, we should have a pretty good idea at this stage just what the real cause of the problem is.

After we are sure we have the cause isolated, it's still a good idea to take a quick check of past history. Did this same thing cause the same problem at some other time? Have we had this same problem caused by a shift change or cutover to new equipment before? Have we always had this problem when we put in new equipment? There are a couple of good reasons for checking past history when we have identified the causes. First, has someone identified this as a cause before and tried to solve the problem by eliminating the cause? Did the problem go away? Did it turn out to be more expensive to solve than the solution was worth? Did it turn out to be only part of the solution and the rest made the problem just as bad? Are the basic ingredients still there; that is, the same people, the same location, the same equipment? If they are, did the solution just fail to take effect or has something else—some new ingredient—entered into the picture?

The second good reason for checking history is to find out if there is any history of the problem *going away by itself.* Some problems are that way. When there is a change in the housekeeping routine, trouble develops. Supervisors know they should do something but aren't sure just what. Then, before they know it, the problem has disappeared. The danger in this kind of thinking is that most of us tend to expect that *all* problems will go away sooner or later. This just isn't so. Many potentially good supervisors have fallen by the wayside waiting for the problems to disappear. Even many problems that seem to leave come back in another form—often a much more horrible form. So we can't wait just because some problems do go away. But we can find out if this particular problem is caused by this particular thing that has a history of repeating itself, then going away. For example, when it's time to replace a typewriter in the office, we can be sure that there will be someone who isn't happy with your selection of who gets the new one, no matter how fair your decision is. (Employees don't always want fairness—they sometimes want new typewriters!) A check with supervisors who have been around for a while will tell us what to expect when the new typewriter decision is made. This same check may tell us that it's all right that some of the typists are miffed; they always are, and it will wear off by itself. If we are satisfied that this is right, and that the new typewriter caused the problem, then we can be equally satisfied that time will heal the problem just as well as any other solution we pick. Of course, if we know enough about the situation before we select the new typewriter or the person getting it, we may do some things to keep the problem from arising.

FINDING THE ALTERNATIVE SOLUTIONS

Now comes the tricky stage where we have already determined the cause and are going to try to find the best solution, the solution that will eliminate whatever is causing the problem. The reason this is tricky is that it is the last time we can really use much imagination or ingenuity. What we want to do now is to think of several possible solutions, not just one. We want the *best* one, and there is a way of getting it. The process is to *brainstorm*; that is, to think of as many alternatives or options as possible without making any efforts to evaluate them, or decide on one, or throw any of them out as not being feasible. The most important thing is to be sure not to allow ourselves to think "Well, I'm sure that won't work, so I'll rule it out now." About the only rule is to concentrate on those solutions that will most likely remove the cause we have located. If there is doubt, *keep the idea around* anyway, unless the doubt is very strong. (We might even ask ourselves "Why did we think of this in the first place? There must be some reason it came to mind, so I'd better keep it for a while.")

The problem with evaluating too early is that we may rule out some good ideas by just not getting around to thinking about them! We hit on an idea that sounds good and we go with it, thereby never even thinking of alternatives that may have been better in the long run. To make it worse, the idea we picked to solve our problem may end up by not being as good as we thought, either because it has some flaws in it, or because it wasn't as practical as it had sounded to us in the beginning. By the time we find it out, we may have used up too much time or gone too far to consider other options. We may even find ourselves committed to this one and have to support it knowing it isn't the best possible solution to our problem.

After we have spent some time listing (either mentally or on paper) all the ideas that we can think of, we should take a last look at them and see if anything else comes to mind. This will tell us if we've paid too much attention to just a single line of thought. Often ideas cause us to think of other ideas, so the time may be well spent. By the way, this is a good place to ask "When do we know when we have enough options to choose from?" The answer is that we have to look at the problem and decide *how much time it's worth*. The bigger the problem, or the more complex it is, the more time we can devote to solving it. Two things are sure: we can spend too much time by just going on looking for more alternatives, and we can be pretty sure that we will reach the saturation point on productive ideas after a while—in other words, we reach a point when the same amount of time no longer produces the same quality of alternative.

An advantage of listing the options we have looked at is that at some point when we are trying to justify the solution we chose, we can say, "Well, I considered these other options but here is why I chose this one." If we have done a good job of thinking out our decisions, we can show why the way we took is better than the ones we rejected. Of course, if for some reason there is a need to take one of the other options (company policy, budget considerations, etc.) then it's also good to be able to say, "I considered that also, and if we go that route, then here are the things that will have to be done...." A final advantage is that it's sometimes possible to sell an idea by showing what the alternatives are. If someone doesn't like what we have chosen, it's good to be able to say that the alternatives are thus and so. It's just a lot better for us to list the options than for someone else to ask, "Why haven't you considered this...?'' It weakens our decisions if we have to say that there are things we haven't considered, even if they turn out later to be bad alternatives.

PICKING A SOLUTION

Now that we've gone through all of this, how do we go about picking the best solution from the options we have listed? There are some definite steps and we need to consider them now. First, we need to use a *systematic* approach. It would be a shame to go this far in such a careful manner and then lose all of the advantage by not using the same careful approach in picking the best alternative. The approach should be a screening process to look at each of the options we have picked and see if they meet certain criteria. If they do, we can use them; if not, we can begin to eliminate them one by one.

First, we ask ourselves if the alternative we are looking for is really *possible*. We said earlier that we didn't want to rule out any ideas at that point, but now we start to become more critical. Now is the time when we decide whether or not the idea will really work. Is it within the capability of our group, our talents, our budget?'' Even if we have the capabilities, will it really work under the conditions that exist in *our* work situation? Will our people accept the idea? Will this option fit into our way of doing things, considering the routine, our interfacing with other work groups, etc? Then we ask ourselves whether the alternative we are considering is really a *probable* solution. After all is said and done and we are ready to use it, are we willing to stick our necks out and pull for this as a solution? Will the boss accept the idea? In other words, what is the *probability* that the idea will work and will be used? Finally, we ask the obvious question: is the idea *applicable* to this problem at this time under these circumstances?

This last question is the most critical of all. We must be sure that the solution applies to the real problem, the one we finally settled on in the beginning. As we study the alternative to see whether or not to use it, we not only want to know whether or not it applies to the specific problem, but whether it solves the whole problem. We should be comfortable with an alternative that gets this far in the testing, and we will be if we are sure it fits the problem and will solve all of it. Because of the systematic approach we have used, we have eliminated most of the "bad" solutions by now. The way to evaluate the ones that are left is to put them to one more test. We have, of course, placed certain "must" conditions on each of these solutions. Any option we picked had to meet these "musts." But as a consequence, we also find that they meet certain "nice" conditions, some more than others. We have said that we realize that we can't expect everything, but there are things that would be nice to have while we are using the option we chose. One way to pick the best alternative, once we have found those that get this far, is to look at the "nice" benefits we get from each one. Those that meet all of the "musts" and provide the most or best "nice" items become the most attractive to us. It is from this list that we pick the final solution. Stated simply, we pick the one that not only will solve the problem we have stated, but also will give us the best side benefits. We have to be careful here, though, because we don't want to become attached to an idea just because of the side benefits. We end up defending it beyond its merit, when another option might solve the problem just as well, be more popular with other people, and perhaps be the most practical one to pick, *all because of some side benefit we feel so strongly about.*

Once we have chosen an alternative, and this has been checked out according to the suggestions here, we need to state it very clearly. For the benefit of all concerned we should make sure that everyone who hears about the solution knows exactly who is going to do what and what it will take in terms of people, money, and time. If we have decided to move certain people to new locations, we should specify which people, where they will go, and what will be their job responsibilities when they get there. If we have decided to go into overtime, we should state how much overtime will be required, who will work it, and how much it will cost. Remember, early in this chapter we said that this would sound complicated but really isn't—so all of this doesn't have to be put down in elaborate form. It just needs to be available if someone asks. It can be in our minds *if we really have thought out the problem.*

PUT THE PLAN TO WORK

This brings us to the point of getting the solution into being. How do I go about introducing the new idea? Many plans fall through at this point. Again, there are certain questions that must be asked. We have to anticipate problems and try to decide ahead of time how we will handle them. For example, we should consider who will be likely to resist this solution. If we anticipate that one of the senior staff members will try to kill the idea, we should take steps to prevent this, even if it means going to this person and getting him or her to help introduce it or give us some suggestions on ways to make it work. We need to decide what risks are involved in trying this new or different idea, and who will be likely to misunderstand what we are trying to do. How about the department head? Is he or she in agreement? After we've tried to anticipate who will be affected and what problems this will cause, we should see whether all risks, resistance, and resentments are covered. If so, it's time to carry out the plan we've chosen. Before we take that step, we need to assure ourselves that we know what we're talking about. Having gone through these steps should give us the confidence to go ahead with the solution to the problem. We mention this at this point for two reasons: first, the new supervisor isn't always accepted for what he or she knows or does. He or she is still thought of as new and thus not capable of thinking the great thoughts that others with more time and experience can think. While this isn't true, it doesn't keep people from feeling that way so it has to be considered. Second, we should not be afraid to push our ideas. By going through the steps we've discussed, we have become very familiar not only with the problem, but also with the alternatives for solving it. In a way, we have become experts on this small portion of the operation, and this should overcome the lack of confidence that others have in us and that we have in ourselves. This is pretty important to the outcome of the project!

CARRY OUT THE PLAN

Now comes the important part of making all of this work. We have spent valuable time arriving at what we think is the best solution to the problem. We have confidence that it is going to work. But it won't work by itself! If the plan is poorly carried out or not done according to the way we have laid out, the results will make the solution look like the wrong one, even if it's not. Surely the solution deserves as much careful attention in the work stage as it did in the selection and planning stage.

Carrying out the plan means more than just putting it to work, or telling someone else to do the job. It means keeping track of the progress, watching how well things are going, even making adjustments along the way. We must be careful to avoid being so committed to the plan that we can't see things that are going wrong. Our commitment should be to the *job*, not our plan. Again, this doesn't mean that we have to spend a lot of time sitting around watching everything that happens. If we have confidence in the plan, we should be able to let it run its course fairly well. But occasional spot checking should tell us if we are really solving the problem. If we have reassigned some of the workers to different jobs, then we can tell a great deal by looking at overtime figures on a sampling basis. When a work assignment and routine has been changed, then occasionally checking the present results with previous ones will tell us all we need to know about the plan we are trying out.

While we are watching the plan in operation, it's a good idea to keep an eye out for potential trouble. We've already talked about making a note on whether we might expect opposition or misunderstanding. Since we know this ahead of time, we have some good check points. The trick is to know when trouble is brewing so we can head it off, not wait until things are in bad shape before stepping in. The skill of anticipating trouble is a hard but valuable one to learn. It is easier to stop most trouble when it first starts than after it's gone on for a while. If we suspect that someone is going to misunderstand or not like the solution we are instituting, we'd better make sure that they don't get too many opinions formed before we deal with their misunderstandings. It will be a lot harder to change their minds than it will be to help them make up their minds in the first place.

Part of the reason for watching the progress of our solution is to check on our own problem-solving ability. We will need to know—sometime in the future—just how well we did at defining the problem, selecting alternatives, and picking the right option. Not only will we want to know how well we did at this, but we will want to get a look at the value of the solution. As we think about our future problem-solving efforts, we will want to ask ourselves, "Was all of this done efficiently, or did I spend a lot of time coming up with a solution that is now falling apart at the seams? Further, did I do a poor job of anticipating where the trouble would come from?" All of this leads to the final step, that of following up on the solution after the plan has been put to work and all the smoke has cleared.

FOLLOWING UP ON THE SOLUTION

The simple question we ask now is, "Did the solution really work?" The answer will tell us most of what we want to know. No matter how well thought-out the plan was or how well we implemented it, if it didn't solve the problem, it really wasn't very good. But if it worked and we got the side benefits we thought we would get, then we'd have to say that the solution was a good one. If possible, we should try to find out why the solution worked. This may seem strange, but there is always the possibility that the problem disappeared in spite of what we did, rather than because of it. All this means is that we look and try to determine whether other factors were at work at the same time which may have had an effect on the outcome of the problem-solving effort. While this isn't worth a lot of time, it's worth at least a little to keep us from getting caught thinking we have solved a problem by ourselves when what someone else did had as much to do with the outcome as what we did.

As mentioned earlier, we should always be looking for flaws in the solution. How could we have avoided the less desirable things that happened? Were there obvious signs that we missed, or was the error unavoidable? Would it have been worth the extra time to look longer for possible trouble? This is simply hindsight, but it's valuable. It can help us avoid making the same mistakes twice. It can help us measure our own ability at problem solving. It can be of help to future problem solvers, because if we have a good idea of what happened, they can learn from both our successes and failures. Of course, all of this presupposes that the problem is dead, not just sleeping. Sometimes problems disappear for a while just because we have done something different; then, as soon as things settle down, they creep up on us again.

Part of following up on the solution includes finding out just exactly how much it took to make the solution work. How much did it really cost? How much overtime did we really put in that was directly related to our solution? Is the job actually more complicated as a result of our action? These are fair questions to ask, and we may well need the information to support our next idea. If we have exceeded our estimated expenditure, it's a lot better that we, rather than someone else, catch it. Also, when we find out exactly what the costs were in terms of money, material, and people, we can honestly answer the question, "Was it worth it?" This can be done only when all the facts and figures are in.

CONCLUSIONS

In the beginning of this chapter we said that the process seems complicated. What we have tried to do is give the complete layout for an approach to problem solving. It will be a rare day when we use each of these steps in its full extent. No matter. The idea is to see that the approach to problem solving is systematic, not haphazard. Breaking it down into steps, as we have done here, shows more clearly that there is a beginning, a middle, and an end. The middle is only one step—picking a solution. What comes before and after determines how well the solution we pick is going to work. Briefly, here are the steps as they have been given:

1. Defining the problem.
2. Gathering the information.
3. Finding the cause of the problem.
4. Finding alternative solutions.
5. Picking a solution.
6. Putting the plan to work.
7. Carrying out the plan.
8. Following up on the plan.

It wouldn't hurt us to write these down and paste them somewhere around our desk. When we start on a problem to

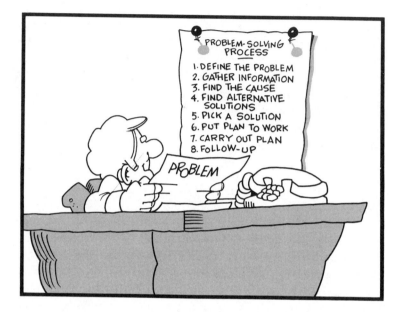

solve, we can take a look at the list and check where we are
right now in the problem-solving process. If we can't decide
where we are, we'd better not be too confident of our solution.
But if we're lucky (or just happen to be doing a good job), we
can find out exactly where we stand in the process and continue in full assurance that we're heading down the right road.
We should have no fear that our solution will not be the right
one!

THOUGHT QUESTIONS

1.   Which of the eight steps in the problem-solving procedure
     is most often neglected in your hospital? Can you see any
     way you, as a supervisor, can help overcome that weak-
     ness?

2. How can you train your staff to use the eight-step approach to problem solving?

3. Problem solving in a hospital always means "change" to someone. How do you get people to change their behavior in your hospital?

4. How can the technique of brainstorming be used in the problem-solving process?

Unit III

SUPERVISORY ACTIVITIES

Chapter 10

Interviewing

While it is unlikely that as a new supervisor you will be asked to make the final decision about hiring someone to fill a position, there is a good possibility that you will at least be asked to interview the applicants. Interviews are held for a variety of additional reasons, such as counseling, discipline, appraisal, and employee termination. You will probably be involved with at least one of them almost every day.

The purpose of these various types of interviews is to predict, change, or identify behavior. In an employment interview you are attempting to predict behavior; in a disciplinary interview you are trying to change behavior; in an appraisal interview you are concerned with determining exactly what an individual's behavior is and evaluating it.

BASICS

Basic to any of these interviews is the need for the supervisor to make the person he or she is interviewing feel comfortable. This is often difficult to do because of the environment in which the interview takes place. It is not uncommon for a supervisor to have no official office, to share an office, or to use

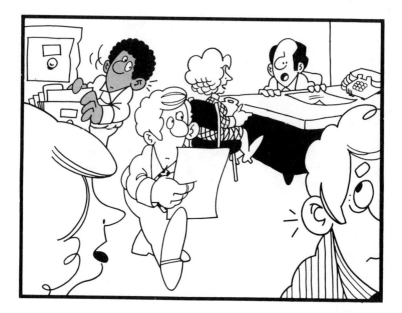

conference rooms or a nursing-station office that doubles for
other purposes. In cases like these it can be difficult to insure
privacy and to conduct a relaxed interview. Nevertheless, the
ingenious supervisor who can anticipate about how long it will
take and whether or not the interview will necessitate privacy
can often make the proper environmental arrangements.

It is important for the subject of the interview to feel that
the procedure is being conducted fairly and that the supervisor
is listening. A supervisor can demonstrate concern not only by
appearing attentive, but by later referring to statements made
by the staff person.

Two-way conversation is very important in interviewing.
If you find yourself doing all the talking, try asking some questions that allow you to listen. You may find it helpful to begin
the interview and to help put the person at ease. Trust has to
be established before the interview can really proceed

effectively. Both of you will so react to each other that you either will begin trusting each other or will remain skeptical and unsure. Two-way conversation encourages you to know more about each other so that you can more quickly trust each other.

If you are interviewing a number of people, you will want to ask the same questions of all the candidates in the same way. Allow yourself the complete interview, if possible, before you make any decisions about the candidate. Assume that the person you are interviewing is nervous and that he or she may initially experience difficulty. Try to listen as much as you can since this will show the person not only that you are interested, but that you really do want to know everything about him or her that you need to know before you have to make any decisions.

EMPLOYMENT INTERVIEW

The first few employment interviews you conduct may be fairly anxiety-provoking for you, but you shouldn't avoid developing the skills needed for this activity, since hiring the right person can make your job much easier in the long run. Employment interviews are often taken lightly because they are easier than firings, but many supervisors are endlessly frustrated by employees that they have to keep moving around from job to job and department to department when in fact they should never have been hired in the first place. It's to your advantage to make employment interviewing one of your strongest skills.

The employment interview perhaps more than any other is dependent on two-way communicating. Inherent in it are two decisions that need to be made: yours about whether or not to hire the applicant, and the applicant's about whether or not to work for you. Consequently each of you must offer information to the other. Or, rather, you must take the responsibility both for offering information and for getting it.

First you must offer information. Absenteeism and turnover are higher for employees whose job expectations are not met. Therefore, it is important for you to remember that it is to your advantage to offer as accurate and complete a picture of the job as possible. Too frequently supervisors try to get information without giving it. They try to discover whether the applicant would enjoy the position before they really describe it. Some supervisors try to discuss only the good and pleasant aspects of the position and intentionally leave out the difficult or boring aspects, thinking that if they include these the applicant might not want the job. In reality, the more clearly you describe the job, the more likely you will be to get a new staff person who will stay and do well in the position, since he or she will not be disappointed by any differences between expectations and the reality of the job.

You also need to obtain information from the applicant. It is most important to gain some understanding of his or her past performance in other positions, since past behavior is the best predictor of future behavior. You will want to determine what kinds of promotions and awards the applicant achieved in his or her last job and evaluate his or her work record. Does the applicant stay at a job for several years, or does he or she change jobs every year? You will need a clear description of the skills that he or she possesses. This is of particular concern, since in some areas of the hospital the skills that people have or are presumed to have can literally affect the outcomes of life-and-death situations.

Sometimes in assessing the skills that individuals bring with them, we forget to find out how long it has been since these skills have been used. A laboratory technician who has not worked in a lab for ten years will need a special type of orientation and may only be prepared for positions in which direct supervision is available. Orientation programs are needed for every new employee, but they should be tailored to match the needs of the individual, and this individualization begins with a supervisor who can establish a clear and complete picture of the skills level of a potential employee. It may be that the requirements of one position require someone who is currently proficient at certain skills, while another position may allow time for the candidate to review his or her skills through an orientation and training program.

Finally, gaining some understanding of the personality of a potential employee is very important. It is not enough to know the age and work record of the applicant. Employees who have positions that closely match their likes and dislikes have less absenteeism and less turnover, while extreme personalities—those who are overly anxious or overly driven to succeed—are more likely to encounter difficulties on a job than are moderate personalities. In order to gain an understanding of the personality of the candidate, a supervisor must do as much listening as talking during the interview. Certain open-ended questions can be used to encourage the candidate's communication. Some of these include: What kind of supervisor do you like best? What bothers you most about supervisors? What have some of your good supervisors been like? To determine how the candidate gets along with other people, a supervisor might ask questions like: Who were some of the people you didn't get along with on your last job? What were they like?

It is to your advantage as a supervisor to hire the right person for the right job. It is also to the new employee's advantage. If persons are not placed in jobs that meet their expectations and fulfill their preferences, they will be dissatisfied and much more likely to be chronically absent or to leave. Therefore, you have a responsibility to both of you to be honest in the decision you make about hiring or not hiring an applicant. Many new supervisors feel guilty but you must remember that you, the new hire, and the hospital will suffer in the long run if the employee is not qualified for the position.

COUNSELING INTERVIEW

As you get to know your staff, they may come to you for help with their problems. Some of these problems may have their origins outside of the hospital, with family and friends. A supervisor should be very careful not to play "psychologist" with the staff, but if someone does have a significant personal problem, then it should be the role of the supervisor to help him or her to get the needed help. It may be that if the employee could talk to a trained therapist such as a social worker for just a few sessions the problem would go away. Occasionally, however, these situations are more complicated than that. Some people are afraid to admit that they have a problem they need help with. They think that it is a sign of weakness or an indication that they are "crazy." This is pure myth, and supervisors should be very supportive of persons in this situation. They should point out that in stressful times like ours it is unusual for an individual never to have a problem of this nature. Certainly most problems go away with time and things work themselves out, but professional help in solving problems can often save a lot of time and months of unnecessary grief. While family and friends can be helpful in times of turmoil, the objectivity and training of the professional therapist can often be more useful in determining the right course to take with the problem.

If a staff person comes to you with troubles related to the job or to the people he or she is working with, the most important thing to do is to listen and to try to understand what he or she really wants. Let's look at an example. Let's say that

Brenda has been working in your department for more than a year. You have been noticing over the last couple of months that she has been late for work a number of times and is quieter and more withdrawn than usual. Yesterday she came back from lunch and was obviously quite upset. She did not communicate with her fellow employees any more than she had to the rest of the afternoon. Today she comes to you to talk about a personal matter. As she enters your office she seems upset and nervous. She begins by telling you that she is having marital problems with her husband, who works nights in a local factory. She then tells you that she has reason to believe that her husband is seeing another woman; she had her suspicions confirmed yesterday. Before leaving your office, she mentions that she wanted you to know what her reason for being late was; she had been waiting for her husband to come home. She also wants you to understand that she had taken care of things, that the problem is under control, and that everything will be okay in a couple of days.

If you were Brenda's supervisor, what would you do? Would you make an appointment for her with someone in the Social Services department? Would you ask her exactly what she meant by "taking care of things?" Would you ask Brenda more about her situation? Or would you be supportive and share with her your sympathy and understanding and leave it at that?

Your role as supervisor is to get the work done, to see that patient services are provided. New supervisors sometimes get too involved with the personal problems of their staff, and these problems then tend to become an excuse for not getting the work done or for poor quality work. Supervisors need to let employees know that they are genuinely interested in them, but that they will respect their right to attend to their own problems so long as they don't interfere with the job. Brenda's tardiness, however, is something that should legitimately concern you, and you need to share your concern with her.

In reality, Brenda's supervisor told her that he was very sorry for the pain she was experiencing in her personal life, but that it sounded as though she had taken positive steps to correct the situation. He explained that he trusted that she would be able to see the problem through, though he also offered to make himself available to listen to her if that would be helpful, or to provide her with a referral to a counselor if she felt that would be useful. The interview ended with Brenda feeling that her supervisor had listened and understood, even though he had told her that he expected her personal problems not to interfere with her work or that of the rest of the staff and that her tardiness would stop. She felt as though he had offered his help and was genuinely concerned.

When someone comes to you with a problem, listening to what they are really asking for is very important. Our usual response when someone is in trouble is to want to DO something. This can undermine an individual's attempts to solve his or her own problems. Often what people need is to be told that they have good problem-solving skills and that in the past they have handled more difficult problems and you feel confident that if they feel they are on the right course, they probably are. Certainly referrals, when appropriate, should be made. But by automatically making a referral or telling someone what to do, we are saying that we don't feel that person can solve his or her own problems and that we know what is best.

The last thing to remember in a counseling interview is that you must be especially careful about what you write down. If a staff person comes to you and requests to talk in private, you need to make very clear whether or not you can provide a confidential relationship. Data of a personal nature should never be put in someone's file, where others have easy access to the information. Individual hospitals have policies about these types of situations, and you should be aware of them in advance of having to use this information with a member of your staff.

DISCIPLINARY INTERVIEW

One of the most difficult activities you will have as a new supervisor is your first disciplinary interview. It can be difficult for a variety of reasons. Perhaps you genuinely like the person; but no matter what, he does not seem to be able to do his job and keeps breaking the rules. Perhaps it's a staff person that you don't like and you are concerned that maybe you aren't being objective and really giving her a chance. Maybe its someone whom you liked and trusted who "betrayed" you and did something really wrong. Maybe you are particularly anxious because you feel that you perhaps do not have enough data to react to this situation as you should. It could also be that none of us likes disciplining anyone since we all sometimes make mistakes ourselves. But discipline is important because it shows your staff that you care enough about them to react to them when they have done something wrong. Your staff knows that it would be easier never to discipline them, but if, indeed, you say what you mean and follow through with discipline if necessary, your staff will trust you more. But it is never easy to conduct a discipline interview.

There are a few things you can do to make this interview less anxiety-provoking for you. The most important thing is to be honest and consistent and to do and say what you mean. If you have said that you will expect such and such and it is not done, then you need to deal with that situation and with the people involved. But you need to deal with them in a fair and consistent way. Particularly when you are new, your staff will "test" you to see how fair and consistent you really are; whether they can manipulate you, or whether you say a lot of things that you are not prepared to enforce and don't really mean. Discipline is very important, since by disciplining fairly, your staff will understand that you mean what you say, that you care enough to enforce what you say, and that they can therefore trust you.

Preparation for the disciplinary interview should be done quickly, so that the interview can take place as shortly after the event as possible. Still, it may be best to wait a short period of time to allow everyone to "cool off." The person coming to see you needs to know exactly why you have asked to talk to him or her. Some supervisors try to "sugar coat" their disciplinary interviews by beginning with all of the good things the employee does; and in fact some employees may remember only the good things the supervisor said! The more open the concern on the part of the supervisor, the more likely the staff person is to perceive what the difficulty is and what can be done to correct the situation. You should begin with objective facts, since they decrease distrust. You will need to get into the habit of taking notes on poor work or inappropriate behavior, so that when the time comes for a disciplinary interview, you are prepared to validate your observations and concerns with specific incidents that you observed. Some supervisors find it helpful to write anecdotal notes each day on their observations of the person. You must be very careful not to leave these notes "lying" around, and always use an initial instead of a name so the privacy of the individual is protected. Hospitals have specific guidelines about what happens to this kind of data, and it may or may not become a part of a person's record.

It is important that the employees have the freedom to ask questions since this will increase understanding between you. One real problem that many supervisors have is that they do not CLEARLY define what a good job is. How many times have you heard from a supervisor, "No one wants to work hard any more," and from the employee, "You sure can't please the boss no matter how hard you work." If you attend to the employee's questions and feedback, you may find that you need to identify more clearly what you consider a good job to be.

APPRAISAL INTERVIEW

Appraisal interviews are often required yearly for all hospital employees, but a good supervisor will not wait that long. Periodically, you should meet with your staff for an appraisal of their work. This is an appropriate time to praise good work. It also is a time to define clearly for the individual what your expectations are for his or her performance. Those supervisors who show concern enough that they will hold short interviews with their staff to ask them what their goals are and to plan for training and developing new skills will experience less absenteeism and turnover in their staff. Later we will be talking more about your role in meeting the training needs of your staff, and we will look at establishing a contract with an individual on the staff for improving or developing skills in a particular area.

EXIT INTERVIEW

Some hospitals require an exit interview, and others do not; but it would be good for the new supervisor to schedule an exit interview with all employees who are leaving, even if it is not required. Since you have to work through others as a supervisor, you will want to be aware of all of the factors that may influence their performance. One of the best places to collect this data is from a staff person during the exit interview. If an individual is leaving because of unhappiness, it is very helpful if he or she can tell the supervisor specifically what caused the dissatisfaction. Was it the pay, promotions, the size of the hospital, the type of supervision, the people he or she was working with, or a job that did not meet his or her expectations or that was too repetitive? Maybe you as the supervisor did not make clear what exactly the job was and what you considered a "good" job.

The exit interview is not a time for argument or for complaints about everything in general. If employees know that your interest is genuine and that (for whatever reason) you really would like their comments on the factors we have just described you may get some very valuable information from them. Your support during the interview will increase their willingness to talk. You should also spend more time listening than talking, though it is helpful to ask questions that will bring out information, such as "There must have been some good things and some bad things about your job here. Can you describe what was the most satisfying and the least satisfying aspect of your job?"

DEVELOPING INTERVIEWING SKILLS

A helpful way to evaluate how you are doing in conducting your interviews is to evaluate each session at the end of the interview. You have already planned the reason or goal for the interview—predicting, changing, or identifying behavior—and now you should evaluate whether or not you have met those goals. Try asking yourself the following questions:

- Did I plan it well?
- Did I put the employee at ease?
- Did it go as I planned?
- Did I really accomplish anything?
- How did the employee feel when it was over?
- How did I feel when it was over?

Again, as we've encouraged you before, if you experience difficulty in this area, identify your area of limitation as clearly as possible and then seek out help from a professional trainer or your department head for help in further developing your interviewing skills.

If I had it to do over again, would I do it differently?

THOUGHT QUESTIONS

1. As a new supervisor, you are preparing for an appraisal interview with a long-term employee who has a mediocre work record with the hospital, but who has remained on the staff without evidence of efforts to change the situation. What would you do?

2. What ways can you provide regular performance-appraisal interviews for your staff to avoid the "only-once-a-year" trap?

3. Sometimes staff members reveal problems in counseling interviews which a supervisor is not capable of handling. Where in your hospital would you refer your employees for help with these problems?

4. Make a list of things you should do before one of the interviews, and try using it as a checklist for the next few interviews you conduct to see if it helps as a refresher, reminder, and guide.

Chapter 11

Training

One of the biggest mistakes supervisors—new and old—make is to assume that training is an adjunct to their regular job, something they do only when they have plenty of time and nothing else to do. An attitude like this indicates that the supervisor doesn't really understand his or her job very well, since the real function of the supervisor is to get work done through other people. Taking this another step, we can say that the supervisor's prime job is to see that his or her people are trained. If a supervisor has anyone who can't do the job because they haven't been trained, then the supervisor has fallen down on the job as far as that person is concerned. Unless his or her people are properly trained, the supervisor has no real justification for appraising them, or for finding fault with their work. Training, then, becomes an important part of the supervisor's job. The new supervisor will do well to learn how to train others if he or she expects to succeed as a supervisor.

TRAINING: A SUPERVISOR'S ACTIVITY

Unfortunately, there are many people around who want to classify the ability to train others as an art or a science. Maybe it is, but it is also a skill, and like any other skill it must be learned. Sometimes we go in the opposite direction—we tend to think of training others as something we can do without any special skill. After all, we say, what's so hard about telling or teaching someone how to do something we know all about? The problem is, that's what we usually do and call it training—we "tell" someone how to do it, and telling isn't training.

There are many skills supervisors have to learn. They must learn to write, speak, conduct interviews, and train their people. Unfortunately, they can do these things in such a way that it will appear that they are doing all right when actually they aren't. We watch someone doing some training and it looks and sounds as though they are doing a good job, but we may be fooled by what we see and hear. The person being trained may not really get the message and may go away frustrated. The person doing the training may think he or she has done well, and go about his or her business thinking the employee should do the job satisfactorily. Later we may hear the trainer say, "Don't you remember, I told you last week how to do that?" The point is that the employee gets the blame for the poor job of training done by the supervisor. So we must learn how to train; that is, we must learn the skill of training others.

There are some things we can put off learning, but training must be learned very quickly if we are to get the most work out of our people. Not only must we learn how to train others quickly, but we must learn how to do it well. Every time we do a poor job of training someone, we waste time that can't be recovered, and we also get ourselves into the dilemma of not knowing whether to train over again or let the employee go on doing the job only half well. The truth is, we rarely repeat the training, but we do end up spending a lot of time trying to repair damage done by poorly trained employees. The worst thing that can happen, of course, is that we end up blaming the employee for not being able to do his or her job, when we've really failed at ours.

But we can learn the basic skill of training others, if we recognize it as a skill and work hard at learning it. We cannot assume that just because we know the job we're training the employee to do we also know how to train someone on that job. Operating a respirator is quite different from *training* someone how to operate a respirator. There are steps to training that we can identify and measure. We can tell whether or not we have done a good job, and we can improve on the skill once we learn what it is that makes up the skill. Let's take a look at the skill in more detail and see just what it is that makes up this thing that some want to take for granted.

WHY TRAIN?

If we ask whether training is necessary, the obvious answer is, "Of course." But if we ask why we train, we get some strange answers. Some train just because there is money in the budget. Others train because the employees expect it. There are those who train because administration has decreed that it be done. Others train only when they have spare time, then they train to fill up the time. None of these are reasons for training. Basically, there are only three good reasons for training.

1. The employee can't do the job.
2. The employee can do it but not well enough.
3. The employee is doing the job incorrectly.

In the first case, not being able to do the job, it may be that the employee is new and has never done it before. This is an obvious case for training, but there are those who say, "Experience is the best teacher—let them learn the hard way as I did." This isn't a very practical approach from the standpoint of patient care or services. Maybe the employee will be better able to do the job after he or she has made numerous mistakes, but who pays for all the mistakes? Who "unlearns" for the employee all the things he or she has learned to do incorrectly? If the employee is new, then for his or her benefit and that of the hospital, it's our job to see that he or she has an opportunity to start off learning the right way to do his or her job. Only then can we get an accurate picture of how well he or she is performing and progressing. But it may be that the job is new, never having been performed before by anyone in the organization. It may be a new procedure or a new piece of equipment. Here, again, the employees have a right to get started on the right foot. Also, for the good of the new policy, let's get the job done correctly from the beginning. Anytime we introduce something new there will be enough problems without us complicating things by doing a poor job of training.

The second case—training because the employee can't do the job well enough—isn't quite as simple as the first case. It may be that the employee hasn't been trained and has picked up some of the job on his or her own. We need to speed up his or her work output and save on wasted time. Now we are faced with the question of whether or not to train because, after all, the employee knows something about the job already. We have to weigh the time and expense of training against the advantages of doing the job faster or better. The same is true even if the employee actually had some training at one time, but needs more in order to meet the standards that have been set ahead of time. We have to decide how much it's worth to get the improvement we can get from training.

Finally, there is the employee who is actually doing the job incorrectly. This is valid ground for training. How do we know the employee isn't able to do the job? We may be able to tell just by the number of errors that can be traced directly to that individual. It may be that a survey of some kind has caused us to look more closely at each employee and we see that this one is failing to do the job correctly. It may even be that watching the employee work quickly convinces us that he or she actually doesn't know what to do. This sounds like reason enough for training, but we need to ask ourselves one basic question before we do any training. "If the employee's life depended on it, could he or she do the job correctly?" If the answer to this is "Yes," then training isn't the answer; there is some other problem, and training won't solve it. So when we train, we must be sure to ask ourselves for what reason we are training; to enable the employees to do the job; to enable them to do it better; or to enable them to do it correctly. We need to ask this question for each employee we train.

This all sounds simpler than it really is. If we aren't careful we'll find ourselves training someone who has had the training some time ago. To compound the problem, the employee's performance may even improve for some time right after the training, especially if he or she enjoys getting away from the job for a while. But the chances are good that he or she will just do poorly in the training session and go back to the job wondering what kind of a supervisor we are to repeat training he or she has already had. Even worse, we end up giving training a bad name; because the employee can't do the job any better after the training, some will conclude that training is a waste of time.

Another possibility for error is to train someone who isn't really going to have time to apply what is being learned. Maybe the employee is just a few months away from retiring or moving to another job. Everyone else on the floor has had the training so we schedule this employee for it also. It's fine to worry about our employees' feelings, but if we train someone simply because we don't want to hurt his or her feelings, we need to remember that it's also our job to worry about the hospital's money. How can we justify spending training money when it's obvious we can't get our money back from an employee who won't be on the job that long?

There is another time when it is a mistake to train: when we train an employee we want to see promoted. We don't train because he or she needs it or because he or she can do a better job for us, but because it will look good on this individual's record if he or she has had this particular training program. Unless this is a part of the employee's regular development program, we've made a mistake when we train for this reason. The problem may come to us in a strange way; it may happen that we have set a precedent that anyone who takes this kind of training expects to be promoted, or everyone wants to be sent to the training program because they think it's the way to move up. In either case, we've put an undue burden on the training program and asked it to do something it wasn't intended to do.

Finally, one of the things that helps us get into trouble is training someone we know hasn't got a chance to learn the job because of his or her background or lack of experience. Some supervisors send certain people to training programs to prove a point—that the employee is incompetent. Again, we've used training in the wrong way, and have failed to do our job properly; we have failed to train the right people for the right reasons.

PREPARING TO TRAIN

Before we can do any training of our own, we must determine just what it is we want to train the employee to do. What are the training objectives? This sounds simple enough, but it really isn't. For example, we should be sure we know exactly what standard of performance we want the employees to achieve. This means analyzing the job to make sure we can train someone else to perform according to the established standard—that is, to do the right thing in the right time with no more than the acceptable number of errors. The standard isn't what someone else has done on the same job that we thought was pretty good. It's not what has come to be accepted as the average for employees doing this particular job. It's what the hospital has set as a standard for the job itself. We need to learn to set job standards by looking at the work, not at the employees who are now or have been doing the job.

Before we train, we'd better get policy questions settled, too. We'd better find out if there are changes in the mill that will make our standards wrong. If there are acceptable deviations from the job standard, we'd better know about it before we start to train. There's no reason to be afraid to ask questions about standards, because we can never be sure that our training has really been done properly if we don't know what the standard actually is. Remember, many so-called standards exist only because everyone has accepted them without question—maybe even perpetuating error or mediocrity in the process. This is particularly true with things like work flow. For instance, just because file cabinets were once put in a certain place, business office insurance records flow around them, even though it would be more efficient to move them closer to the verifiers who need them. As a result of this poor arrangement, the work has suffered, but the "standard" has been set. If we don't watch out, we'll find ourselves training to this standard. We find this to be true of such things as admission forms and charge slips, too. We try to train someone to fill out the complicated form or charge slip without ever questioning why the form is so complex. The truth may be that it got that way because every once in a while someone added something to it without trying to cut out anything. Pretty soon it became unwieldy, but we keep on using it as the standard and trying to train people to use it. A few well-chosen questions might help "uncomplicate" the forms. In fact, just listening to our employees might help. They probably know that some things are unnecessary, but no one has ever bothered to ask them. Remember, they are doing the job, so no one else can be more familiar with what is actually being done than they are. If we can't come up with a better reason for doing something or not doing it a certain way, we should take their word for it.

It's highly unlikely that we can ever train for everything that needs attention, so we have to decide early in the game just what it is we are going to include in the training program for each of the employees. For example, if the employee is new on the job, we should concentrate on those things that will be likely to come up first in his or her new assignment. It will be enough to do to learn the things that must be done immediately without worrying about things that will come up several months from now. If the job is being changed, we should concentrate on the changes, not the entire job. It's wasteful (and boring to the employee) to go through procedures that the employee already understands. Even after we have decided what to train our employees to do, we should still check and see if there are any existing programs that will do the job for us. Maybe someone on another unit already has some kind of program that will come close enough to doing our job for us so that it wouldn't be worthwhile for us to develop an entire training program to make up the difference. It's always well to check this out before going too far. By the way, we mustn't forget to check with other departments about their training programs. Sometimes we get so out of touch with others in the same hospital that we don't even know that they have the same training problems that we have and may be conducting programs very similar to the ones we are preparing. We ask ourselves, "Why hasn't someone done this kind of training before?" Then we ask, "Who else has the same kind of training problems I do?" The answers to these questions should help us screen what's available well enough to prevent us from inventing the wheel all over again.

Once we've decided what training needs to be done and why we're doing it, we must set some realistic objectives or goals for the training we are going to do. The simplest way to do this is to ask, "What is it I want them to be able to do when the training is over?" Basically, the answer to this question depends on the answers to the following ones:

- What is the action I want from them?
- What is the standard I plan to use to gauge their success?
- What are the limitations or tolerances I can live with?

If we've taken a good look at the job as we suggested earlier, these things should be clear by now. We should know what a satisfactory job is, and if we don't, it will show up when we attempt to answer these questions. It's not enough just to say, "We want them to understand how the data terminal works." We have to specify the action and the degree of tolerance we expect to allow. Requiring that a central supply clerk package 100 items an hour with no more than two errors is much more specific than requiring an understanding of how to use the machine. One reason training is so haphazard is that we go about it in a haphazard manner. We just suddenly discover ourselves doing some training without much real planning. When we do a sloppy job of planning, we do a sloppy job of training. The planning doesn't have to be elaborate or time-consuming. A plan can be written out on the back of an envelope, but it should be done. We need to decide where the training is going to take place, just who will be trained, and when it will be done.

DO IT RIGHT

It seems ridiculous to say it, but when we train, we should do a good job of it. As silly as it sounds, though, we find that some training is better than other training, hence some people are doing a better job than others. The reason is that we don't always know a good training job when we see one. Supervisors can be heard to say, "Don't you remember, I told you...," which means that they think "telling" and "training" are the same thing. In fact, when we watch them "train," they end up doing most of the talking and the showing, then leave with a statement like, "Any questions?" The employees think they understand, the task looked simple enough, but after the supervisor leaves, the employees find that they can't really do the job after all. They feel pretty stupid because they've just seen the supervisor do it, heard an explanation, and didn't have any questions—*all because the supervisor did a poor job of training*. Since training is a skill, we can't expect to be good at it right away. We can try to learn the skill, though, and as we do more and more of it we can evaluate the results and grow with it.

Good training follows specific steps and procedures. When we train people on the job, what we do will have a definite bearing on how well they can perform in the future. The most accepted process to use is a simple, three-step one that has worked well for many years. It goes like this:

Step 1
We tell them what to do.

We do it correctly.

Step 2
They tell us what to do.

We do it correctly.

Step 3
They tell us what to do.

They do it correctly.

Notice the purpose of each step. In Step 1, we tell the employees what is to be done so there will be no doubt about the action and so they will be mentally involved. Then we do it correctly, being sure they see each part of the procedure. In Step 2, they are still involved mentally as they tell us what to do; and if they tell us correctly, we do it correctly again. In Step 3, they tell us what they're going to do, but do not do it until we have agreed that they are right. If they are, then we let them do it. Step 3 can be repeated several times for practice, but it's always a good idea to keep the employee involved mentally as much as possible. After all, this is where the memory is established. Even though we want the employees to develop good work habits, we still want them to perform from a good mental attitude. To increase this mental involvement, we can expand the three-step process to include not only what, but why and how. We still go through each step as described above, but after going through what, we repeat the process by telling how. Then we repeat with why we perform the operation the way we are doing it. In other words, the first time through we simply worry about the employees seeing, hearing, and doing the right thing. They see how, but we don't go into it in much detail. Then we repeat the process, this time adding a description of how we do it—so that they hear a description of the correct way to perform the procedure, while doing it. Finally, we go over the what and how, but add to it the reasons why we use a certain movement or tie it a certain way, or move the ribbon to the left.

It should be obvious that when we are doing this kind of training, we have the employees use the actual equipment, or something that looks just like what they will be using. Ideally, they should be trained on the equipment they use every day, right at the spot where they do the job. If not, then we should try to find idle equipment that is like what they will be using. As a final alternative, we can use something that closely simulates the regular thing they use, but we should remember that the less imagination they have to use, the better they will be trained. If they get dirty on the job, they should get dirty during the training. If they write on blue paper on the job, they should have blue paper during the training. By the way, there's a simple point that is often overlooked: in training, never face the employees; always demonstrate to them from

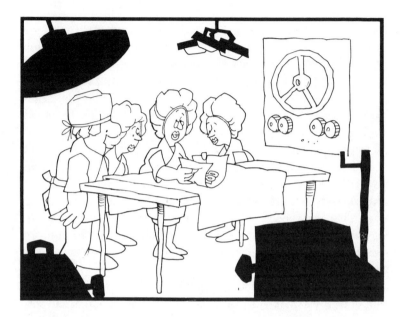

the same position they will take when they do the work. If we face them, they will see everything done backward and may become quite confused when they try doing it themselves.

FOLLOW UP ON TRAINING

One final word about training: we shouldn't just train and go off and leave it. We should follow up on what we have done and see how well the training "took." Training is more than doing it, marking the training record, then forgetting about it and the employee and saying, "Well, that job is complete." We should go back to the employees and see how they are doing. Check their performance against the standard we set. Check error rates, look at outputs, see if the secretary's letters are better—check the results of whatever the training involved. If the employees are performing well, we can take credit for a job well done. If not, then we need to take a look at our procedures to see if we failed to do the job properly. The rule in this case is simple: if the employees are doing something we trained them to do, we are responsible for their performance until we find out that something other than their training is keeping them from doing the job. Of course, we are always responsible for their performance in a way, but now we look for some other cause because we are satisfied that the training has been done correctly. If we follow the proper procedures, we can be sure that the training has been done correctly.

In addition to training, you need to be aware of your staff's need for continuing educational opportunities. This could be in the form of a course, or workshop, or institutes. These may be either outside of the hospital or programs designed within the hospital. Your staff need to be encouraged to stay up-to-date in their particular technology. You too need to be aware of and try to provide for your own continued growth. It's important!

THOUGHT QUESTIONS

1. Recall instances in which new equipment or procedures were introduced in the department, when more training or better attention to training would have eliminated the problems that existed. How would you have done it?

2. What kind of training should a new supervisor have? What retraining should be given to that supervisor when he or she needs it? How do you know he or she needs it?

3. We've talked about formalized structured training at length. What other effective approaches or methods of training would you use as the supervisor?

4. What does the statement "workers and subordinates should help train their supervisors" say to you?

5. How does a supervisor train and retrain in good safety practices?

Chapter 12

How to Run a Good Meeting

As a new supervisor you may find yourself feeling as though you are doing nothing but going from one meeting to another. The need for meetings could be debated forever, but the problem is not so much whether or not to have meetings, but rather how to make them effective. As a new supervisor you should begin to develop good conference skills to help you improve the quality and effectiveness of meetings for which you are responsible.

PURPOSE OF THE MEETING

As the leader of a meeting, you should begin by looking at the purpose for the meeting. This is important, because the purpose will influence your role.

Frequently in hospitals we use "brainstorming" or *idea-generating* meetings. For this type of group it is important that everyone be kept involved. Andre Delbecq has developed a technique called the "nominal group," in which you first ask every group member to spend ten minutes writing down all of the ideas or solutions he or she can generate. Then, as leader, you begin writing ideas from each person's list on a blackboard

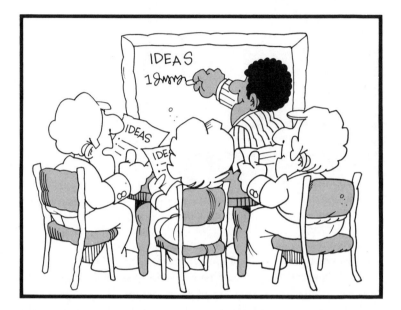

in round-robin style. Take everyone's first item, then the second, and so on. As the leader it is your role to encourage everyone to participate but not to tell the group what to contribute.

Another type of meeting is for *judgment and evaluation*. These meetings are best in smaller groups so that decisions can be reached by consensus; that is, by determining where all members of the group agree instead of by voting for or against an idea. The size of this group is best limited to from five to seven people. As a new supervisor you will not only lead this type of group, but you may also be a member in a group that has to make some very important decisions based on the group evaluation of a situation. An example would be a hospital faced with a situation in which it could not raise daily room rates, but in which each department had to determine how it could cut costs and still provide quality care. The supervisors in each department need to make some important judgments or decisions based on their evaluations of the situation: do we reduce our staff or some of the services we provide? The role of the leader in this situation is to discuss each issue throughly and not allow the group to average, or vote, or resort to some other shortcut. It is necessary that all supervisors reach a consensus, because facts and logic rather than argument are very important in this type of group. The supervisors then return with the decisions made in their meeting and lead an *informational* meeting with their employees, in which they exchange and disseminate information.

The informational meeting is a third type of meeting. There is a distinction between disseminating and exchanging information. Sometimes, as a supervisor, you will be meeting with your staff to disseminate information. Usually in these types of meetings, you will clearly control the communication, which will flow in one direction only. Sometimes, however, you will be asked to meet with your staff and to tell them something that requires exchange of information. In that case it is your role to make sure that all parties are heard from and that there is a climate conducive to exchanging information. For example, a housekeeping staff may be brought together to be told by their supervisor that painters will be painting all the rooms on the psychiatric unit during the week. The group should discuss how this will affect their daily work activities and exchange information on how their work can best be accomplished under the circumstances. They may decide that certain cleaning activities would best be postponed until the evening shift.

The last type of meeting groups can have is an *attitude development* or "pep talk" meeting. In these kinds of groups, the leader should be active in determining what he or she wants accomplished in the group and should actively participate in the accomplishment of these goals. It is very important for the leader to find out what people in the group want and then link their needs to the accomplishment of what he or she wants. For example, if you want your staff to change their daily schedule to accommodate a special assignment, try to discover what the group would view as a reward, and see if you can link your goal with their needs. If you want them to view the upcoming celebration of the hospital's anniversary with enthusiasm and support, perhaps it would be helpful if you could arrange for the staff to have the afternoon off, providing that they come in an hour early to help with the setting up of the displays and not take a lunch break. This is the most effective way to handle the "pep talk" type of meeting. Rarely are you able to influence the attitude development of a group through persuasion and argument alone!

SUGGESTIONS

Once you have determined in advance the purpose or purposes of the meeting, have provided for the appropriate types of activities, and are prepared yourself for the role you will assume in each, what next? *Publish an agenda.* Remember, it is necessary to define for your staff what a good job is. By publishing an agenda you are giving the group a road map so that they will know what they are supposed to do. Also, by having an agenda you can decide what type of activities or role you should accept for yourself. Perhaps one of the items on the agenda should be brainstormed, while another requires judgment and evaluation and a consensus needs to be reached. Thus, an agenda is very important.

Publish a written record of the meeting.   In groups decisions are made, information is given, and policies are initiated and discussed. Unless there is a written record, these outcomes may be misinterpreted or forgotten. In addition, we tend to forget those things we have accomplished and to remember those things we have *not* accomplished. By having a written record, we remind the group of what they have accomplished, so that they don't get absorbed with what they have not accomplished.

Start the meeting on time. As a new supervisor, it is particularly important for you to start the meeting on time. When we talked about testing we mentioned coming late, whether to work or to a meeting, as a way of testing an individual. If you wait until everyone has arrived before starting, or if you start even a little late, you are rewarding those people who come late, and this is undesirable. It is very important to reward good behaviors, rather than persuading people to change or punishing undesired behavior. So don't punish the people who are on time, reward them. Also, do not review or summarize for the people who come in late; require them to seek information from the people who were on time. When your staff realizes you really mean it when you say two o'clock, eventually they will begin arriving on time. One supervisor, whose staff did a great deal of testing by coming late, got into the habit of starting on time and dealing with the most important topic first. The staff soon realized that the most important part of her meetings was the first few minutes and made a habit of being there on time. Another reason you should start on time is that this is another way that the staff can learn to trust you. They are learning that you mean what you say; and therefore they will feel as though they can trust you, since you do what you say you are going to do.

State the ending time at the outset. The group members will work more efficiently if they know in advance how much time they have. In addition, there are some group members who need to know the target time of completion as well as the goals or agenda of the group, because they work best in those kinds of group situations. On the other hand, do not be tempted to make the meeting longer if the group has not accomplished its goals. If you have told the group that they need to decide on two issues in an hour, your role, after a half hour, is to remind the group of the goal and their progress. The group may test you to see if you really will end on time, so make sure that you do what you say. If the group has difficulty dealing with a problem and really needs more time, the leader should ask the group before the time is up if they want another meeting or prefer to lengthen this one.

Preschedule regular meetings.   When meetings are held on a regular basis, schedule them in advance so that you can manage your time and your staff can manage its time most efficiently. "Spur of the moment" meetings should be used for emergencies only. Remember, though, if the meeting is scheduled in advance and there turn out to be very few items on the agenda, consider cancelling the meeting. There is nothing worse than a meeting for meeting's sake!

Consider the specifics.   As the leader, ask yourself, "What specific activities will take place?" This is important in terms of the arrangement of furniture, the reservation of equipment, the selection of rooms, and so on. The activities will determine whether you will need to seat everyone in a circle, provide tables, or just set up chairs facing the front. But you need to know more.

You should decide on the "specific timing" for the meeting; that is, not just how long it will run, but what day and what time of day. If it is to be a one-hour meeting, try not to run it at a time that would usually conflict with an established coffee break. On the other hand, if it is to be a lengthy meeting, providing for a break in the middle might be a good way to inject some relief. Having meetings at the tired end of the day or week, when everyone is thinking about going home, is not the best time to get into brainstorming sessions. Don't run long meetings into the lunch hour or quitting time, since if the group needs more time, you will automatically have to call a new meeting.

Lastly, you need to know the "specific attendance," not just how many are going to attend, but who is going to attend. There is always the consideration of seating, including who sits where and how many seats will be required. You will need to look at who should come to the meeting. If it is to be a group where you make judgments and evaluations, the number of individuals needs to be kept to a minimum. If such is the case, you need to have enough people there to represent everybody concerned without weighing it with too many people from the department who support one side of the issue.

PHYSICAL FACILITIES

The place in which a meeting is held is very important. If the room is poorly ventilated, too hot or too cold, the purpose of the group may be difficult to achieve. You need to consider the creature comforts, the acoustics, visibility, and interference when evaluating the physical facilities in the room, and this should always be done in advance. The room should be comfortable; the members should be able to hear and see each other; and there should be no outside interference, such as a running dishwasher or remodeling going on.

HOW TO CONDUCT A MEETING—OR CONFERENCE LEADERSHIP

There are three stages to every meeting, and as a new supervisor you might want to try identifying these stages in every group you are in, whether as a member or as a leader. The first stage is the *initiation* stage. Typically it only lasts a few minutes, though in some meetings it lasts longer because there are group problems. The goal of the initiation stage is for all of the members either to meet each other or to become comfortable with each other's presence, to learn the purpose for the meeting, and to meet the leader and perhaps test to see if he or she is to be trusted.

As the leader of the meeting you should position yourself at the head of the group. This encourages the members to see you as the leader. Next, you should anticipate that there will be some noise and commotion initially, so do not begin the meeting immediately with your most important message. You might want to say something like, "Well, let's begin. The purpose for today's meeting, as you can see by the agenda, is. . . ." This allows time for the group to settle down and to begin paying attention to you. Once you feel you have the group's attention, identify the reason for the meeting and try to get some feedback from the group. Encourage participation whenever possible, since you want them to be able to "test" you and come to trust what you say. For example, after the agenda is discussed, ask the group if they are in agreement with your plans for the meeting. If you pause and allow a little silence, the most anxious member will usually break the silence and begin to give you some feedback. However, it may be too soon for their engagement, and you may need to go on and discuss one of the topics before the group will begin participating. How familiar the group is with each other, how often they meet, and how large they are will, to some extent, determine how long it will be before you can encourage active participation by the members and move into the second stage. In very large groups, it may be almost impossible to encourage participation. The ideal size of a group for the maximum amount of group process is five members.

Remember that your anxiety will be high at the beginning of the meeting. You may interpret silence as a sign that you have done something wrong or that you aren't doing a good job, or you may be tempted to call on people to participate. You should recognize that these feelings are NORMAL and that the best procedure is to go on with the meeting and give the members the time they may need. The best way to deal with these initial feelings of anxiety is to anticipate them and to try to prepare yourself well for the meeting so that you will be confident. Some new leaders try to begin a meeting by saying something that will indicate sympathy with the other members. Never try to "impress" the group with your intelligence. If you do, the group members will just wait for you to make a mistake, and then they can disagree with you. You want them to listen and participate in the meeting instead. Anticipate some testing such as members challenging what you are saying or your right to say something or perhaps even the need for the meeting. But do not become defensive. This is a normal occurrence at this stage of the group, and you should deal with it as you do all types of testing—with consistency and honesty. Be firm, but considerate and consistent in the way you respond to the testing behavior. The group will discover by the way you respect the challenging member but still set limits that you can be trusted—that you say and do what you mean.

Occasionally, you may encounter a group that has difficulty moving into the second phase of a meeting. The members may continue to test you and "not get down to business." There may be a "hidden agenda" in this group. In other words, perhaps members have come wanting to use the meeting for another purpose. If such is the case, you may have to vocalize your frustration to the group and ask if they are aware of any reason why moving on is difficult for them today. If you find yourself consistently in this situation, you may want to ask someone to come and attend a meeting that you lead to see if he or she can help you recognize the problem.

The second stage of a meeting is the *working* stage, in which the goal of the group is to accomplish the purpose for the meeting. We have already discussed how this might vary from problem solving in judgment and evaluation groups to brainstorming in idea groups. This is the most productive part of the meeting, and the smaller the group and the more familiar they are with each other, the longer this stage will last. In newly formed groups and in large groups, this stage is usually relatively short. If it appears that the group will not be able to complete its business in time, do not wait until the group enters the termination stage to ask the members to decide whether they will extend the meeting time or will meet again to finish their business. If you wait until they are in the termination phase, you may get a hasty decision, or you may encounter some reluctance to meet again.

The *termination* stage, the last stage, is often short and is characterized by many of the same social behaviors as the initiation stage. The goal of this stage is to prepare people for the end of the meeting. People will start getting their belongings together and will make commotion just as they did as they were getting settled in the initiation stage. You may find the group becoming more social and even testing again, perhaps challenging either what has been accomplished or your role as leader in terms of implementing some of the decisions made during the meeting and so on. Again, anticipate this behavior and do not interpret a "bad" last few minutes as an indication that the whole meeting was bad. This type of behavior is normal and is not necessarily related to you at all. All groups end this way. Remember to end on time and to conclude by summarizing. Never try to accomplish any work on the purpose of the meeting when the group is terminating. This is usually very frustrating, and the quality of the work achieved is usually poor.

COMMON GROUP PROBLEMS

There are three common group problems. The first one is conflict within a group. This frequently occurs when the task of the job is impossible and the members become frustrated. Or it may occur because the group members are loyal to conflicting interests or are more interested in status in the group—that is, who is most powerful—than in what the task of the group is. There may be conflict because the members are really involved in the task of the group and they feel a real commitment to the decision the group makes. This conflict, however, is usually constructive rather than destructive.

The second common group problem is apathy and non-participation. This can occur when the group members feel that the purpose or task they are working on is not important or that they would prefer working on another problem. But even if the problem is important to members, there may still be underlying factors that lead to apathy. For example, if the members fear being punished if they make a mistake, they may do nothing. Other reasons for nonparticipation are feelings of powerlessness about influencing final decisions, or a prolonged, deep-seated conflict among a few members of the group which dominates the group process.

The last common problem in groups is inadequate decision making. Often making satisfactory decisions is a major struggle for a group. This is especially common if a decision is called for prematurely and the group has not achieved cohesiveness. It may also be that the subject may be threatening to the group, either because of unclear consequences or fear of reaction of other groups.

We have discussed the importance of determining the purpose for the meetings you are to lead. We have made some suggestions about how to prepare for the meeting and how to conduct the meeting. We also discussed some of the common group problems. But how do you actually learn to lead a group? You will learn by doing. Your hospital may provide you with training programs in group skills and techniques if you request it, but the best way of learning how to lead a group is to do it and to evaluate yourself continually. Ask yourself, did I meet the purpose of the group, and if so what did I do to facilitate the purpose? If not—why not? What was the problem, and what else should I have tried doing? What will I do the next time to avoid the problem or, if it should occur, how can I deal with it differently?

THOUGHT QUESTIONS

1. Your department head wants all supervisors to meet with their staffs to discuss some recent problems in the area of patient relations. He or she is anxious for everyone in the department to display the proper concern for the importance of patient-staff interactions. How would you prepare for this meeting, and what role would you assume in the meeting?

2. If you need a small, representative group to meet and make some judgment about a policy decision, how would you decide whom to ask to join the group? How and when should physicians be invited and involved in hospital meetings?

3. You are leading a meeting in which the purpose is to decide on the vacation schedule for the year. You are in the process of discussing how the group will decide who will get first choice if there is a conflict, when two aides and a nurse get into a verbal fight. How would you handle this situation? During what stage of the meeting is this most likely to occur? Using the information in this chapter, what could be the reason for this type of group behavior?

Chapter 13

Oral and Written Presentations

As a new supervisor, you will be expected to begin making oral and written presentations immediately. These may range from the informality of memos and small discussions to formal letters and speeches. Taken together, they form the basis for the flow of knowledge in the hospital. Later in this chapter, we will offer a few specific guidelines for each of these, but there are some basic rules that apply in general to all good oral and written communications. The preparation of any communication should begin with a consideration of your subject matter, your audience, and yourself.

Knowledge of your subject may be your strong point. Many new supervisors have been promoted to their new position because of extensive knowledge in the area. Others, however, may have been promoted because of leadership and organizational skills and may need to work very hard at quickly developing knowledge in their special areas.

Whatever your situation may be, never rely on luck or your gift of gab to make up for a lack of knowledge. As a supervisor, you must know what you are talking about if others are to trust you. In addition, you are an important role model for your staff, and unless you want them to begin operating on misinformation and half-truths, you must make certain that you are as well informed as you can be. This does not mean spending weeks in the library, but it does involve preparation time. It is not expected that you will know everything, but your staff will be able to tell whether or not you are prepared. They will also appreciate your honesty if when you have made an error or do not know something, you feel secure enough to admit it and to do something about it.

You must also know your audience. When you write a memo to or address a specific group of people, you need to know them well enough to anticipate how your message will be received. You need to plan carefully to gain their interest and to avoid speaking over their heads or confusing them. And if the message is controversial, you will need to be very careful with the words you choose, since there may be some hostility involved and you will want to present your message as clearly as possible.

Finally, you must know yourself. We have emphasized many times in these chapters that good supervisors know their own strengths and limitations and work to develop the skills they need. They do not just let things come as they may. If you are aware that you have difficulty with written communications, then set about improving that very important skill. The same is true for oral presentations.

BARRIERS TO GOOD WRITTEN COMMUNICATIONS

Probably the most common barrier to good written communications is the habit of sending out insignificant memos. How many of them have you received and read in the last week alone? If you want your staff and your fellow supervisors to read your memos, send them only when they are important and necessary. Many supervisors bombard their staff with written communications in an effort to keep them informed about changes that are being made. The result, however, is that a staff will very quickly begin realizing that most memos are not important and then will stop reading them altogether. If you must use this method to keep your employees informed, it would be better to organize these small messages and publish them together once a week or once a month.

A second barrier is hiding important messages within others. Consider the following memo:

To the staff on Units 3W, 4N, & 4S

It was a pleasure to have Dr. Lipson visit us last week. He seemed very impressed by some of the changes we have made on the units, and he assured me that we are on the right track. As you know, I am anxious to use outside consultants whenever they can help us. I also rely heavily on your input into the areas we should be working on to improve care on our units.

As a result of Dr. Lipson's visit, I will be reevaluating each job description and collecting data for possible reclassification. I will be meeting with you individually and in small groups within the next month.

Again, I would appreciate your input into our new endeavors and also what you thought about Dr. Lipson's visit with us. Some of you have mentioned that it was particularly helpful, but I would like to hear from everyone.

D<small>OROTHY</small> J<small>ONES</small>, R.N.

If you were a staff member on this unit and just glanced at this memo in your pay envelope or posted on the bulletin board, you would probably miss the implication that major changes were about to happen that could potentially affect your classification. This memo not only hides that announcement, but is vague and unclear as to why it is being done, who is going to be affected, and when it will be implemented. You as a new supervisor should learn to write memos carefully and

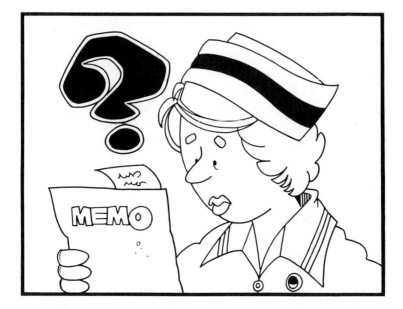

if necessary have someone read them for clarity before sending them out.

Another pitfall to avoid is sending messages so that you can say, "I sent a memo." Messages sent for ulterior ends can only fail and may reflect badly on the person who sent them. To be effective, written communications must directly express the reason for which they are being sent.

The last major barrier to effective written communications is the use of slang or jargon that others may not understand, and this can be an especially serious problem in the hospital. Take, for instance, this memo sent to the Director of Purchasing by the evening Head Nurse:

> We need a different type of H-clamp. The handles on the ones we have are too long. I've marked the length on a pair so you can see. It's next to the crash cart inside the treatment room. (That's the room across from the room

where we put all the T & A's). Thanks for taking care of this for me.

Unless the personnel in Purchasing happen to be very familiar with "H" clamps, crash carts, and "T & A's," this memo is going to have to be followed up by time-consuming phone calls or additional memos. That sort of wasted effort can be avoided by using language appropriate for your audience.

GUIDELINES FOR WRITTEN COMMUNICATION

Good written communications begin with a decision about the purpose for sending them. There are three reasons for writing letters or memos: to communicate information you have to someone else, to request information from someone else, and to substantiate or document something in writing. Once you have decided whether you are writing to inform, request, or document, you will be better able to find the right words to use for your purpose.

Second, open your letter or memo with a brief statement of its purpose. The most important parts of a written communication are the first line and the last line. You do not need to be blunt or tactless, but you should tell your reader as quickly as possible what the communication is about. For example, introductory sentences like "Here's the answer on the incident report that you asked for" are much clearer and convey the message much more quickly than do lengthy introductions and explanations leading up to the subject of the communication such as this:

Due to employees who were on vacation, and because of a heavy production schedule in our department for the last few weeks, I haven't had much information for you; but here at last I have the information you asked for.

Once you have told the reader what your communication is about, you can go into detail. Again, however, your basic purpose is to communicate; so avoid jargon and obscure phrases that may not be familiar to your reader.

Finally, end your communication with a sentence that contains what your reader should do or know. "Take the necessary steps to secure a bid on this for us," leaves the reader with a concise message that is hard to miss.

You develop good writing skills by writing, so practice, reread what you have written, and continue writing. It may be very helpful to find someone who is a successful communicator and to study his or her style to discover what it is that makes his or her writing precise and easy to read.

BARRIERS TO ORAL PRESENTATIONS

We all have experienced nervous speakers, whether it be in small discussion groups or in formal lecture situations. Their anxiety is contagious, and an audience may have a difficult time concentrating on the presentation. Your own personal discomfort in making an oral presentation may be the biggest barrier to getting your message across. Dealing with anxiety is basic to effective oral presentations. You may find that it is easier to speak in front of a group when your self-esteem is high, perhaps after your department head has praised you in front of everyone, because your confidence is increased and you feel good about yourself. However, you aren't always going to be able to schedule your presentations when you are feeling good. You will have to learn to accept the fact that how you feel will affect your presentation and do your best to minimize the effect it has. If you are feeling low, you might engage in something you do well prior to making your speech.

A second barrier to effective oral presentations involves your sense of presence as you face your audience. Speakers who slump over a microphone or who tap the table vigorously as they talk tend to distract their listeners from the message. If you use a microphone, adjust it to the right height (or at least know how to adjust it), to make certain that your audience can hear you. If you have notes, be careful to avoid rustling the papers. And if you have a pager, you should decide beforehand whether or not to turn it off if you want to avoid being interrupted. The key is to avoid distracting your audience through unnecessary motions, noise, and interruptions as much as possible. Your purpose is to get them to concentrate on the message you are trying to communicate.

The last barrier to effective oral communication is being unresponsive to the audience's reactions. You need to be aware of their response to your presentation, and in fact they can make your job easy. If they are alert, smiling, and friendly, you're doing fine. If they look bored, sleepy, or hostile, you may need to call for feedback from them. Ask for questions or a vote or some other type of response to engage them in what you are saying. And try talking *to* them and *with* them rather than *at* them.

GUIDELINES FOR ORAL PRESENTATIONS

As a supervisor you will be asked to present a variety of oral communications. It may be to address new employees as part of an orientation program or to present a report on how to conserve energy in your department at a meeting of other supervisors. Or you may be called on to address the public and press about some recent event in the hospital. Each type of presentation requires its own preparation, but you must begin with a consideration of the basic rules of knowing your subject, your audience, and yourself.

When you are preparing your speech and have done your research and know what you want to say, begin organizing your material by making note cards. You don't need to write down your entire speech, just the phrases and statistics you want to be sure of remembering.

Secondly, begin preparing for your speech at least a day in advance by practicing it using your note cards. You should work on your words and phrases and try different combinations of phrases to get the most out of the language. Practicing opening remarks is particularly helpful since that will be the time when you will be most nervous. If you get off to a good start, you will develop confidence as you go along. It may be helpful for you to practice in front of someone, to make sure your presentation is logical, clear, and understandable. It is very common to be vague or confusing without realizing it, and a friendly listener can often help you avoid giving a weak presentation. Remember, if you are doing poorly it is a sign that you need more practice, not a signal to stop doing it altogether.

Finally, you may want to consider the use of visual aids. People remember what they see and hear much longer than what they just hear. Visuals can also save you a lot of words. However, if you are considering using a visual aid such as a chart, slides, videotape, or overhead projector, make sure that you get help from someone who knows how to make and design them, so that they will be effective and versatile. And if you do use visuals, remember to arrive early and to check out the equipment to make sure that everything you need is there and in good running order.

HOW TO DECIDE WHETHER TO HAVE A MEETING OR SEND A MEMO

Sometimes you will find yourself in situations in which you will have to decide whether you will use oral or written communication. Consider the following example.

You are the new Pharmacy Supervisor and you have just been told about some changes in payroll policies that will affect your staff. You now have to decide how best to communicate this to everyone on your staff. Your choices are: (a) speak to the staff in small groups on each shift, (b) pass around a memorandum to all of them, (c) appoint several to come in and get the message and then take it back to the rest of the staff, (d) post the message on the main bulletin board near the door to the pharmacy.

In common situations like this, you need to consider the advantages and the disadvantages of each method. There is no right or wrong way. Every situation needs to be evaluated individually. If you consider (d), the disadvantage is that some bulletin boards contain everything from announcements about missing dogs to cars for sale. You have no assurance that all employees will see it, unless you go around and remind everyone to look at it. The advantage is that it is very efficient and uses very little of your time. If you consider (b), you need to be aware that when a memorandum is passed around it has the advantage that everyone gets the same message at the same time in the same words. The disadvantage is that if there are questions, your staff is likely to ask questions of each other rather than of you. Calling in a small group of leaders, (c), has the advantage of letting you use the leaders on your staff to go back to the others and do the selling of the information for you. The disadvantage is that the information can become distorted, since it will be coming from several people instead of just one. This disadvantage can be minimized by having the staff go back with copies of the memo to be passed out as they relate the information. The final approach (a), speaking to the staff in small groups on each shift, gives you the advantage of being available for any questions; and it may also give you some feedback and an opportunity to work through any resistance that you encounter in the staff related to this information. The disadvantage is that it is very time-consuming.

SUMMARY

Because of the complexity of activity in the hospital, the flow
of information through oral and written communications is
essential if you, your fellow supervisors, and your department
head are to be able to achieve the goals of the hospital. In addition, it is desirable for supervisors to be available and supportive of their staffs and to represent their staffs to others fairly.
With this in mind, you should begin a program to develop your
oral and written skills; these skills are necessary if you are to
be supportive and fair in the way you deal with your staff, as
well as able to communicate information to others in the hospital.

THOUGHT QUESTIONS

1. Policy and procedure changes occur frequently and
   rapidly in the hospital. This means that you are probably
   deluged with communications about these changes. What
   approach would you take to combat the five barriers discussed:
   a. Hiding important messages among unimportant ones.
   b. Sending insignificant messages.
   c. Sending messages for ulterior motives.
   d. Poor organization of the message.
   e. The use of slang or jargon others may not understand.
2. What can you do to assure feedback from the messages
   you send?

Chapter 14

Self-Development

It would be easy to stop the book at this point with just a few words of exhortation about personal growth and development. But the new supervisor needs to know how and where to develop. As we become embroiled in the everyday problems of the job, we forget to look at ourselves to see if we are any better at what we're doing than we were a few months ago. In fact, we forget just what the areas are in which we are supposed to improve. Little problems seem like big ones when they are with us, so we spend all of our time worrying about them and fail to realize that a good supervisor has to think about the future as well as the present. Not only do we need to worry about the long-range objectives of the hospital, but we need to think about some long-range objectives for ourselves. This isn't to say that we should spend all our time worrying about the next job or our "big promotion"; we simply have to realize that we really aren't going to be of much value to ourselves or the hospital if we fail to grow to our full potential. But how do we develop ourselves, and what are the areas that get first attention? The answers to these questions will make the difference in where we will be ten years from now and what we will be doing then.

HOW DO WE DEVELOP?

How can we improve ourselves if we have all the problems of the job to worry about? The chances are that we are going to be so busy we can't take time out to train ourselves, or even do much planning about the future—and here we have the first indication that we need some development. If we can't get the job done in the time allotted to us and still find some time to look to next week and next year, we may need to look at the way we are doing our job. Are we really organized in our work effort? Are we spinning our wheels doing things that should be delegated to others? Are we doing things over because we aren't doing them right the first time? Are we spending too much time on small, insignificant details, thereby letting problems get bigger and bigger? There are some pretty good signs to look for to see how well we are doing. Let's see some of them and what we can do about them.

First, the matter of not having enough time. One sign that we aren't utilizing our efforts very well is that we are working without taking time to plan. It's a vicious cycle, because the less time we have, the less we plan; and the less we plan, the more time it takes to do the job, so we run out of time. This goes on and on until finally we discover ourselves swamped with work and no time to plan it. The results are that we don't do a very efficient job of what we do, and may even overlook doing things that should be done. But how do we get out of such a dilemma? We must turn the process around by stopping the cycle. We can start this by taking even five minutes at the start of the day to try to put things in order. If we don't do this, we'll probably do the first thing that comes up, whether it's important or not. Five minutes of deciding what needs to be handled first and what will wait will save us from getting behind on important things. Another five minutes will allow us to decide what we need to handle and what we can delegate to someone else. Another tell-tale sign that we need to watch for in our supervisory job is the tendency to justify doing more and more of the job ourselves "... because I can do it in less time than it takes to explain or train someone else." When we get into this cycle, we're doing more and our people are doing less. They're not happy because they see us doing work that they could and should be doing. We're unhappy because we're doing work we shouldn't be doing, and may even decide that our people are lazy or have a poor attitude because they aren't doing more—all because we haven't taken the time to plan our work very well.

Remember, these are indicators that we need to develop, not solutions. The matter of how we develop is just as important. So far, we've seen that one way is to force ourselves to do five or ten minutes of planning and delegating. Another way is to give ourselves a little "instant success." We need confidence in ourselves, and this comes from accomplishing something. Even if the thing isn't the biggest or most important job we've ever done, just finishing a task—and stopping long enough to take note of it—will help our confidence a lot. How can we use this technique to our advantage? One simple method is to make a list of the things we have to accomplish in a period of time: a day, a week, or two weeks. (If our confidence is fairly low, a day works best.) We list the things that need to get done today. We can make another list of things that should be done sometime in the near future. During the day we mark them off one at a time as we complete them. A good way to mark them off is with a transparent felt-tip pen. This way we can see what job we did, and that it has been accomplished. Seeing the broad strokes of the felt pen gives us a boost, because we see that as hectic as the job has been, we've still accomplished a few things. The next day, or at the end of the day, we make a new list, taking the things done off the list and adding new items for the upcoming day. Two things become pretty obvious as we follow this procedure: one is that it shows us how much we are really doing, and the other is that it gives us excellent chances for planning and organizing our work. As we see the things we have to do, we may see some duplication of effort. We may see that someone else who works with us can do two or three of the items because of the close relation between them. Also, as we list the things to be done, we have a chance to set some priorities. Naturally, we want to do the important things first, so they should be near the top of the list. To avoid procrastination start with the least desirable task first, while we're still fresh, instead of at the end of the day. Also, complete one task before starting another. One caution here: getting the right "size" is important. Writing down something that's going to take two or three days isn't going to give us much confidence; it will have just the opposite effect. If we see the list is short and each item takes a day or more, we need to list some of the parts of the job that can be done separately, and then cross these off as we accomplish them. This, too, helps us organize the large tasks into small, logical steps, helping us do a better job overall, and still giving us frequent "successes."

Another way we can develop is to watch others. First we watch our boss or someone else who is getting a lot of work done in the same time we're working. We study their behavior, their pattern, their organizing. We try to figure out what it is that makes them able to get as much done as they do. We can even discuss the subject with them. Don't make it a "flattery" session, though. They probably get a lot done because they make good use of their time; we don't want to be guilty of taking up too much of their time with our poor organizational habits. The way to discuss the subject is by asking the right questions, not by asking the person to solve our problems. We watch the person work, then ask why he or she did certain things. "Why did you call the meeting right at that time? What advantage did you gain by having the meeting at all?" Of course, we need to make it completely clear that we aren't questioning his or her wisdom, just trying to improve on our own. To improve on our perception, we can try to anticipate what the answers will be. We try to figure out the reasoning behind what was done, then see how close we were to the reasons he or she gives. As we get closer and closer, we can see that our judgment is getting better. We're probably making better decisions on our own job now.

THE NEXT JOB?

There are two reasons for developing ourselves—to do better in our present job, and to be ready for the next one. It is important to keep them in this order—the present job, then the next one. This may sound simple enough, but many good supervisors fail to be promoted because they get so interested in the next job that they forget to deal properly with the present one. They think, talk, and plan about the job they hope to get, letting the details of the present one slip. The first thing that happens is that their interest also begins to wane and pretty soon disaster strikes. An important assignment gets only meager attention. Details are overlooked and wrong decisions are made. Errors creep in and higher management gets involved in finding out what happened. The poor supervisor, who was potentially able to take on more than he or she is now assigned, is found to be losing some of the work he or she used to have because someone up the line doubts this supervisor's ability to handle even the present job. Some have said, "Do well on the present assignment, and the future will take care of itself." That's pretty good advice, except that it doesn't include all that's necessary to get ahead. It assumes that the things that are needed on the next job are already in the present one. This may not be true. If not, then it's well to develop in those areas where we are weak. If the next level above us requires consider-

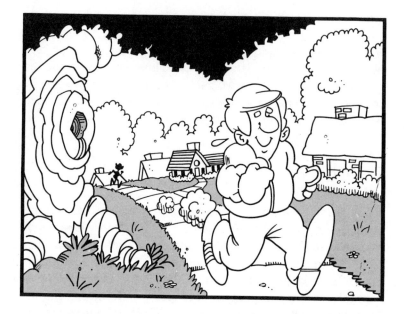

able report writing and we don't think we're very good at it, this is one place we can start. We can look around for places to learn more about report writing, and we can look for opportunities to do some report writing on our present job. We can start off by making short reports on things the department head has asked about, then work up to longer and more complex ones. Just doing reports is a good way to learn, but we should do some studying and developing on the side so the experience will be meaningful. We follow the same routine in the other areas where we think the next job exceeds our present requirements. The advantage of this approach is that it will actually make us look better on our present assignment, rather than making us look like we have abandoned any interest in it. While we are improving in our existing job and improving our reputation at the same time, we are also preparing ourselves to take over a more responsible task when the opportunity arises.

One final word: think enough about yourself to spend time on yourself. Spend some time doing what you like. Read books and magazines. Take night courses. Do something for yourself. Begin a vigorous exercise program or learn how to meditate. You certainly are aware of the fact that you have taken on more responsibility with your new position, and with that comes more stress and conflict, more anxiety and depression. You should begin to develop new habits to handle this increased stress.

Strenuous exercise programs, those activities that make you huff and puff, exercise your heart too. Many supervisors have found that in addition to the value to the heart, such exercise also gives you more energy each day and will help to reduce stress. You will find yourself sleeping better and having more energy.

For an exercise program to work and to offer you genuine benefits, you must engage in it for 20 minutes at least three times a week. It is important to develop an exercise program slowly and with a physician's supervision. It should also involve something that you enjoy. Some people jog, others swim, some play handball or go bike riding. Whatever your choice, it should be enjoyable and you should think it important enough to yourself and your health so that nothing interferes with your exercise time.

The successful supervisor, new or old, is the individual who is sensitive to his or her own needs for development and will find ways of making the necessary improvements. Perhaps more important than that, he or she will see it as a challenge, not a chore, and will do it and end up calling it fun.

Good supervision can be learned. If we take the time to back off and look at ourselves and where we are going, we'll see that we have already come a long way. It may have been hard work, but that wasn't all it was; there was probably a great deal of pleasure in making the trip. The rest of the way can be even better!

THOUGHT QUESTIONS

1. Making a list of things to do in an identified length of time is a valuable tool for discipline, planning, and personal development. Which people who work for you and with you could benefit from seeing what you put on your list each day or week? Why and how could they benefit from your planning your work?

2. Take the time to analyze the work behavior of a supervisor you admire. What might you learn about supervising from this exercise?

3. Think of an outstanding supervisor you have worked for and jot down those things which you think made him or her outstanding. Which of these qualities are those which you most need to develop further as a supervisor?

4. Identify three critical skills for a good supervisor in your department. What are some of the ways for a new supervisor to develop ability in these skills? How do you tell when you have developed these skills sufficiently?

5. What areas might a supervisor need to be retrained in at some future date?

6. You would like to try an exercise program but you live in an apartment and can't jog in your neighborhood without having to fend off the neighbor's dogs. What else might you consider?

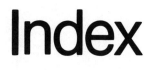

Index

Index